'Back to Health through Yoga, destined  rue modern day classic, is a comprehensive guide to the improvement of one's health through the time-tested path of world's leading authorities on the subject

—AR........, MD, MPH, DYEd
Former Staff Physician: Dr. Dean Ornish's Program for Reversing Heart Disease
Author of *Healing Back Pain Naturally* and *Extraordinary Healing*

'In *Back to Health through Yoga*, Dr. Bijlani has stressed very appropriately that yoga is not callisthenics but a way of life which deals with the body-mind complex.'

—P.K. DAVE, MS, FICS, FIMSA, FAMS
Former Director, All India Institute of Medical Sciences,
New Delhi

'Dr. Ramesh Bijlani has done it again! He has taken up very complex and often misunderstood but very important subjects and crystallized them into very simple and easily understood English.'

—SUDHEER GOGTE, MD, FACC
Cardiologist, Yuma AZ, USA

'Here you have a book by Dr. Ramesh Bijlani, which has all the components which go to make a best-seller, except the hype and the sales pitch. The author brings to bear on his knowledge of the human body and western medical practices, the wholesome perspective of yoga.

'In this book he shows how a healthy life style is a prerequisite to a life which is materially fruitful as well as spiritually rewarding.'

—MANGESH NADKARNI, PhD
Former Professor of Linguistics
Central Institute of Foreign Languages, Hyderabad

'Dr. Ramesh Bijlani is himself on the path of yoga, and at the same time a man with the best of modern medical training. He is not dogmatic, but open in his thinking and outlook. His writing is clear and lucid. His claims are modest and credible.'

—K. RAMAKRISHNA RAO, PhD, DLit
Chairman, Indian Council of Philosophical Research,
New Delhi

'As a new-level integration of health-science and yoga, this book is revealing and reassuring in many ways, remarkable in what it says and how it says it. There is cool confidence and clarity all through. It shows a path, a style of value-added enlarged living, free from mind-body-soul imbalances and disorders.'

—CHANDRASEKHAR RATH, PhD
Former Professor of English, Utkal University, Bhubaneshwar

'Enlightened medical scientists have realized the value of yoga for health, and are attempting a synthesis of yoga and modern medicine. Prof. Ramesh Bijlani deserves appreciation for his contribution in this direction. He has utilized his long experience as a distinguished teacher to put before the medical profession and the lay public the concept of yoga and modern medicine being complementary to each other. Dr. Bijlani has included in his book the management of common lifestyle disorders using this approach, which is fully justified and highly rewarding.'

—B.N. TANDON, MD, FNA, FAMS
Former Dean and Professor of Gastroenterology and
Human Nutrition
All India Institute of Medical Sciences, New Delhi

BACK TO HEALTH
through
YOGA

Dr Ramesh Bijlani is a medical doctor, writer, teacher, scientist, and above all a person committed to using his unique blend of talents for human welfare. Educated at the All India Institute of Medical Sciences (AIIMS), New Delhi, where he did his MBBS and MD, and at the Massachusetts Institute of Technology (MIT), Cambridge MA, USA, where he did a master's course (SM) in nutrition, Dr Bijlani spent nearly thirty years on the faculty of AIIMS, teaching and conducting research on nutrition in relation to cardiovascular disease and diabetes. In 1992, he started going into the depths of yoga, specially the integral yoga of Sri Aurobindo and the Mother. His personal and professional life converged in the year 2000 when he initiated at AIIMS, a patient care facility for providing lifestyle modification courses based on yoga in tune with the latest developments in mind-body medicine. In the year 2005, he took voluntary retirement from AIIMS to find more time for the dissemination of yoga.

Prof Bijlani was elected Fellow of the National Academy of Medical Sciences (India) in 2005 and conferred an honorary doctorate in yoga by Swami Vivekananda Yoga Anusandhana Samsthana, Bangalore in 2006. Besides his research publications, he has written extensively for children, medical students and lay readers – he has twelve published books to his credit.

Yoga destroys all sorrows for him in whom the food, the play, the putting forth of effort in works, the sleep and waking, are all moderate, regulated and done in fit measure.

THE BHAGAVAD GITA, 6:17

BACK TO HEALTH through YOGA

RAMESH BIJLANI
MD, SM, DSc (*Honoris causa*), FAMS

Rupa • Co

Copyright © Ramesh Bijlani 2008

First Published 2008
Third Impression 2011

Published by
Rupa Publications India Pvt. Ltd.
7/16, Ansari Road, Daryaganj,
New Delhi 110 002

Sales Centres:

Allahabad Bengaluru Chennai
Hyderabad Jaipur Kathmandu
Kolkata Mumbai

All rights reserved.
No part of this publication may be reproduced, stored in a retrieval system, or transmitted, in any form or by any means, electronic, mechanical, photocopying, recording or otherwise, without the prior permission of the publishers.

The author asserts the moral right to be identified as the author of this work.

The royalties on this book shall go to
Sri Aurobindo Ashram-Delhi Branch.

Typeset in Sabon by
Mindways Design
1410 Chiranjiv Tower
43 Nehru Place
New Delhi 110 019

Printed in India by
Rekha Printers Pvt. Ltd.
A-102/1, Okhla Industrial Area, Phase-II,
New Delhi-110 020

To
My Spiritual Masters

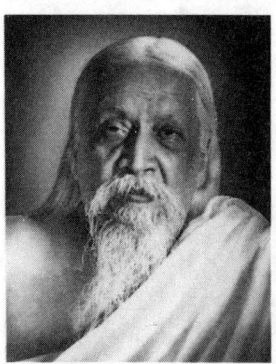

Sri Aurobindo
for lighting the path

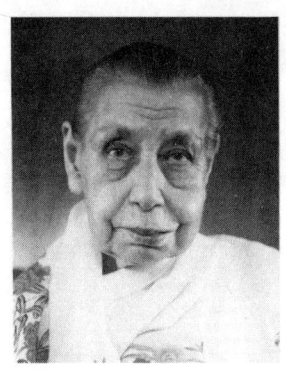

The Mother
for Her abundant grace

Contents

Foreword ... ix
Before You Read the Book ... xi

LIFESTYLE

Yoga: The Finest Lifestyle Ever Devised ... 3
Demystifying Meditation ... 32
Eating Wisely and Well ... 48
All Style, No Substance ... 65
Staying Mobile ... 91
Sweet Dreams ... 113
Don't Worry, Be Happy ... 133

LIFESTYLE DISORDERS

The Mother of Many Maladies ... 153
The Silent Killer ... 174
The Heart of the Matter ... 191
Too Sweet ... 212
Breathe Easy ... 246
The Poor Back ... 260
Gut Feelings ... 298

APPENDICES

Yogic Practices for Lifestyle Disorders ... 322
Words of Wisdom ... 326

DR. KARAN SINGH
MEMBER OF PARLIAMENT
(RAJYA SABHA)
CHAIRMAN
COMMITTEE ON ETHICS

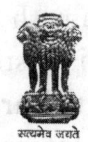

Office : 127, Parliament House Annexe,
New Delhi-110001
Ph. : 2303-4254, 2379-4326
Fax : 23012009
E-mail : karansi@sansad.nic.in

Foreword

Man's ultimate goal is the attainment of a state of perfect consciousness, a state that has been described as divine. Yoga provides a wide array of methodologies designed to effect man's union with the Divine. This system is a gift of our great rishis, who perfected it many centuries ago, and in our land we have preserved this invaluable heritage down through the generations. During the last century, yoga has gained tremendous acceptance throughout the world.

The transition to the state of divinity is through many stages, and the preservation of one's health is one of them. People's lifestyle has undergone drastic changes in modern times, adversely affecting their health in many ways. Yoga is proving to be a boon in coping with the stresses and disorders caused by undesirable lifestyle changes. With the recognition of the mind-body relationship by the scientific-medical community, yoga has increasingly become a part of modern medicine, and doctors are freely advising people to take to yoga.

Any person who wants to adopt yoga would like to understand the mechanism of his own body and the role and correct technique of yoga in relieving him of his disorders. The present book, *Back to Health through Yoga*, by Dr Ramesh Bijlani, goes a long way in meeting the needs of such an aspirant. Dr Ramesh Bijlani, former professor of physiology at the All India Institute of Medical Sciences, New Delhi, devoted himself to learning yoga since 1992. His special interests include the Integral Yoga of Sri Aurobindo and the Mother.

According to Sri Aurobindo, 'All Life is Yoga'. Yoga facilitates the spiritual quest, but this needs a healthy body as well as purification of mind. Yoga can play a useful role in keeping the body healthy. The author has rightly emphasised the importance of the yogic attitude in his book, from which not only lay persons but also members of the medical profession can benefit.

18 May 2007

Karan Singh

Before You Read the Book...

Yoga is not a quick fix for health, but it may hold surprises for those who are willing to make the effort.

KELLY MORRIS

The seeds for this book were sown in the year 2000 when I was instrumental in establishing at the All India Institute of Medical Sciences (AIIMS), a facility which would offer lifestyle modification courses based on yoga for prevention and management of chronic disease. In order to make the courses more effective, I prepared some handouts for the participants. Those handouts have been revised, and several new topics added, and the result is this book.

In order to understand how and why AIIMS, an institution using exclusively modern scientific medicine for patient care, decided to have a facility for teaching yoga, it is essential to go a little at length into the recent history of modern medicine as well as what yoga is. We shall take up both these issues one by one.

Modern Medicine, 1900-2000

Modern medicine made a series of spectacular advances during the period 1900-1950. Several infectious diseases were conquered with the help of vaccines and antibiotics. The mystery of diabetes was solved with the discovery of insulin, and that changed the clinical course of diabetes dramatically. The discovery of vitamins gave a sort of short-cut to the elimination of major nutritional deficiencies. Surgery became safe and painless. Imaging techniques and advances in clinical biochemistry improved diagnostic accuracy to an amazing level. The result was that in Western Europe and North America, which benefitted the most from these advances, the average human lifespan more than doubled. History has been repeated in India after Independence. In 1947, our average life expectancy was about thirty years; today it is more than sixty years. However, while the lifespan has increased, man has not become immortal anywhere in the world. People are now dying at an older age of a different set of diseases, the most prominent among them being hypertension, heart disease, stroke, complications of diabetes and cancer. Grappling with these new killers has been a humbling experience for modern medicine. The advances made during 1900-1950 reinforced our faith in the mechanistic model of life, which is generally traced back to Rene Descartes, a brilliant French philosopher who lived in the seventeenth century. But treating the new killers of mankind on the basis of the mechanistic model turned out to be highly inadequate. The reason is that unlike infectious diseases and nutritional deficiencies, heart disease and cancer are not caused by the presence or absence of a single clearly identifiable factor. Our new disorders are the result of slow accumulation of damage over decades. The damage is inflicted silently in small doses by an unhealthy lifestyle, of which mental stress is a major accompaniment. Accordingly, there began a search for good lifestyles and strategies for overcoming mental stress for prevention and management of disease. Both these explorations converged on the rediscovery of ancient disciplines like yoga which combine superb lifestyles with potent, infallible prescriptions for lasting mental peace. Incorporation of mind-body approaches like yoga into modern medicine was facilitated by a spate of epidemiological, clinical and laboratory studies which elucidated the major role played by mental stress in the causation of disease, and the immense contribution which mental relaxation can make to the treatment of disease. The result was that by the year 2000, the mind-body relationship had a strong scientific foundation. According to Larry Dossey, in 1950 modern medicine left behind the era of physical medicine and entered the era of mind-body medicine. He further explains that while retaining the spectacular achievements of the era of physical medicine, scientific medicine now added to its framework a new dimension based on the mind-body relationship. The new dimension leans heavily on disciplines like yoga. That is how ancient wisdom became a part of modern medicine: the oldest at the service of the youngest.

What is Yoga?

Yoga is a way of life which facilitates spiritual quest. The quest needs a healthy body as well as purification of the mind. How the body may be made healthy, and how the mind may be purified has been worked out over thousands of years by those who have walked the spiritual path. That is why yoga, which is primarily a discipline which catalyses spiritual growth, also gives better health and mental peace as fringe benefits. Far more people are interested in health and happiness than in spiritual growth. Therefore, although yoga is not a system of medicine, some components of yoga may be borrowed by a system of medicine and used for promoting health. This 'trick' is not new. Ayurveda did it thousands of years ago; modern medicine is doing it now.

Yoga and Modern Medicine

Now it should be easy for the reader to understand why, how and in what form yoga has been incorporated into modern medicine. It is not a simple transplantation of a dozen yogic postures: if that were so, yoga in modern medicine would simply be a close cousin of physiotherapy. Yoga is a precious tool in mind-body medicine. The postures, diet and sleep (called physical culture in yoga), meditation (as first aid for stress), and the yogic attitude (for long-term relief from stress) are all a part of yoga, and all these have a place in mind-body medicine. Mind-body medicine aims at correcting the faults in lifestyle responsible for the illness, and thereby creates the best conditions for reversal of the process which led to the illness. It is now known that the body has powerful self-healing mechanisms, which include a well-organised in-built pharmacy. However, self-healing is favoured by right conditions, and the yogic lifestyle is the best way to create such conditions. It is important to emphasise that mental peace and positive thinking are a major component of the conditions for self-healing. People are often quite willing to do a few yogic postures, make some changes in the diet and even give up smoking. These are all good, and do help to some extent. But what most of us do not appreciate is that durable health and happiness also need a shift in the way we look at people, events and circumstances. We can get a lot more from yoga by adopting not just the yogic way but also the yogic view of life.

Closing Thoughts

This book is meant for the intelligent and inquisitive reader who will use it to discover the roots of health and disease. He will find in it reasoned and reasonable guidelines for a healthy lifestyle based on yoga. Stress management has been discussed on the basis of Patanjali's enumeration of the sources of *klesas*. With the yogic attitude these sources of stress simply disappear. Things may not change, but we change in such a way that adversity either ceases to matter, or may even turn into an opportunity for spiritual growth. The major lifestyle disorders have also been discussed individually bringing together at one place our current understanding of these diseases and their prevention and management using an integrated approach that dissolves the barrier between modern science and ancient wisdom.

Although the book has some information on physical practices such as asanas and pranayamas, it is not meant to be a substitute for learning these practices from a teacher. I believe no book can replace a teacher when it comes to physical practices.

In gratitude

I have been very fortunate in that a renowned scholar, Prof M.V. Nadkarni, who is himself a writer, agreed to go through several chapters and made those small but significant changes which make the language lucid, elegant and unambiguous. I have also drawn freely on the expertise of my friends in various medical specialities to make sure that the information is up-to-date and accurate. I am grateful to Prof Manju Mehta, Professor of Clinical Psychology at AIIMS, for going through the chapter on stress management; Dr Rajiv Narang, Additional Professor of Cardiology at AIIMS, for going through the chapters on hypertension and coronary heart disease; Prof Nikhil Tandon, Professor of Endocrinology at AIIMS, for going through the chapter on diabetes; Prof Randeep Guleria, Professor of Medicine at AIIMS, for going through the chapter on bronchial asthma; and Dr Anuj Dogra, Orthopaedic Surgeon associated with Sri Aurobindo Ashram – Delhi Branch, for going through the chapter on back pain. If in spite of their efforts, any errors have crept into the book, the responsibility is entirely mine.

The tedious task of typing the manuscript was cheerfully handled by Mr Satish Sachdeva when I was at AIIMS, and by Mr D.K. Singhal after I joined Sri Aurobindo Ashram – Delhi Branch. The drudgery of proof reading has been shared by my wife, Lovleen, and our daughter, Arpita. I am quite sure there are many more who have contributed to the book in one way or the other; I apologise for having missed to mention them by name.

In Remembrance

For personal reasons, I feel compelled to share with the readers the sad demise of Professor Mangesh Nadkarni, who edited more than half the chapters in this book. Prof Nadkarni, educated at Pune, Hyderabad and University of California at Los Angeles, had taught Linguistics and English at the Central Institute of Foreign Languages, Hyderabad, and the National University of Singapore. An erudite scholar, loved teacher, original thinker, eloquent speaker and prolific writer, Prof Nadkarni had received unique gifts from the Divine, and he used them to serve the Divine through everything he did. He was an ardent devotee of Sri Aurobindo and the Mother, and they had revealed to him the inner meaning of their works as well as given him remarkable ability to put it across. As their untiring ambassador, he travelled extensively, disseminating their philosophy and vision in his inimitably clear style and resonant voice laced with wit and humour. He was on a spiritual quest while also being a householder, which is always a formidable undertaking. He served the Mother till the last breath, and breathed his last in Her lap in Pondicherry on 23 September 2007.

Ramesh Bijlani

Lifestyle

It is only by correcting your ways of living that you can hope to secure good health

THE MOTHER (OF SRI AUROBINDO ASHRAM)

1

Yoga:
The Finest Lifestyle Ever Devised

Yoga is a methodised effort towards self-perfection.
SRI AUROBINDO

The word 'yoga' popularly evokes two contrasting images: one that of a set of exercises/postures (asanas) which are good for health, and the other that of a very demanding spiritual quest meant only for a select few – both the images have some basis in reality. The asanas are a highly visible and rather popular yogic practice, but only a small part of yoga. Yoga is also a spiritual quest, but there is no essential incompatibility between yoga as a spiritual quest and normal everyday life. Ordinary everyday life can be lived in such a way as to lead to spiritual growth. Viewed in that way, yoga becomes a path open to all rather than a practice reserved for a few.

WHAT IS YOGA?

Before coming to what yoga is, it may be better to clarify what yoga is not. Yoga is not synonymous with asanas, pranayama, or meditation. These are techniques which, if practised rightly, can help support the pursuit of yoga. If yoga is not synonymous with these techniques, let us see what it is. To paraphrase Sri Aurobindo, yoga is a journey towards self-perfection by employing systematic effort. It is commonly accepted that man is imperfect, and to be perfect is to be Divine. Hence any movement towards perfection brings man closer to the Divine. Therefore to say that a person has achieved perfection is to say that the person has crossed, or transcended, the limitations of the human state. One might say that he or she has achieved oneness, or union, with the Divine (Fig. 1.1). That is the origin of the word yoga (*yuj,* union). Since the journey towards union with the Divine is long and difficult, it requires systematic effort. That is why most schools of yoga tend to prescribe a system or a method consisting of some well-defined practices or techniques. Spending some time everyday on practising a few yogic techniques such as the asanas and meditation makes it easier to incorporate a yogic attitude into all the other everyday activities. That is how the yogic techniques fit into yoga: as catalysts, as facilitators, but not as the whole of yoga (Fig. 1.2). Thus the techniques are important, but the rigidity frequently associated with them is not.

SCHOOLS OF YOGA

All schools of yoga advocate a movement towards perfection. This perfection may be classified into perfection of the body, perfection of the mind, or that of both. Accordingly there are different schools of yoga.

Hatha yoga aims primarily at perfection of the body. A perfect body means a strong and healthy body. The motto of the All India Institute of Medical Sciences is *sharirmadyam khalu dharma sadhanam,* i.e. right living can be pursued only through the medium of the body. The body is an instrument for all our actions – right and wrong. But in the present context, it is important to realise the importance of the body even for right actions, and here body implies a healthy body. The techniques of hatha yoga include asanas, pranayama and kriyas.

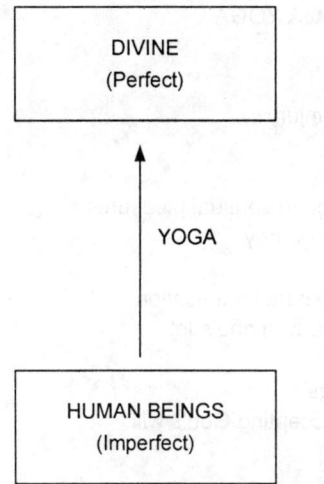

Fig. 1.1. *Yoga is a journey towards perfection, or union with the Divine.*

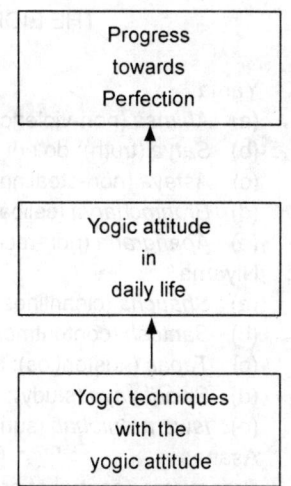

Fig. 1.2. *The role of techniques in yoga. Techniques are means, not the end.*

Raja yoga primarily aims at perfection of the mind. A perfect mind is calm and quiet, and completely at peace. The basic technique of raja yoga is mediation. But since a healthy body can work much better towards a peaceful mind, some asanas and pranayama are also a part of raja yoga. Patanjali, who compiled the classic 'sutras' on raja yoga, divided raja yoga into eight limbs or parts. The first two limbs, yama and niyama are a set of ten dos and don'ts aimed at living a socially responsible and conscientious life leading to self-purification. The next two limbs are asanas and pranayama. The next three limbs are different stages of mediation. The eighth and final limb is 'samadhi', the culmination of all the previous steps, which is achieved only by a select few.

THE EIGHT LIMBS OF RAJA YOGA

1. Yama
   (a) *Ahimsa* (non-violence): do not cause injury
   (b) *Satya* (truth): do not tell a lie
   (c) *Asteya* (non-stealing): do not steal
   (d) *Brahmcharya* (celibacy): do not indulge in sensual pleasures
   (e) *Aparigraha* (non-receiving): do not be greedy
2. Niyama
   (a) *Shaucha* (cleanliness): internal and external purification
   (b) *Santosh* (contentment): being satisfied with one's lot
   (c) *Tapas* (austerities): discipline
   (d) *Swadhyaya* (study): study of scriptures
   (e) *Iswarpranidhan* (surrender to God): accepting God's will
3. Asanas
4. Pranayama (control of prana/'breath')
5. Pratyahara (sensory withdrawal)
6. Dharana (concentration)
7. Dhyana (meditation)
8. Samadhi (superconsciousness)

The yoga of the *Gita* advises approaching the Divine through a combination of work, knowledge and devotion, and yet leaves scope for greater emphasis on one or the other of the three components depending on the temperament of the individual. The beauty of the triple path lies in relying on our three basic instruments – head, heart and hands – for achieving perfection. Use the head to know the Highest, use the heart to love the Best, and use the hands to serve the Greatest.

The *Gita* is primarily a book which encourages action for and in this world. But the *Gita* is over three thousand years old. With the passage of time, a dichotomy developed between worldly life and spiritual life, and this has been reflected in the popular understanding of the *Gita*. In the recent past, Mahatma Gandhi, Swami Vivekananda and Sri Aurobindo have made enormous contributions towards correcting this distortion. Sri Aurobindo's yoga, often referred to as **integral yoga**, is a very powerful synthesis of different schools of yoga. It leans heavily on the yoga of the *Gita* but incorporates the central principles of all traditional schools of yoga. The uniqueness of integral yoga lies in emphasising a few points. First, it considers the world to be not an illusion but a manifestation of the Divine. Therefore the Divine cannot be realised fully or integrally by rejecting the world. Thus integral yoga discourages asceticism. Secondly, integral yoga has its focus on the perfection or divinisation of everyday life. All actions can be divinised, or as the *Gita* says, can be performed with a yogic poise (*yogastha kuru karmani*, II: 48). Finally, integral yoga does not stop at the salvation of the individual. It aims at a collective psychospiritual transformation in ways we cannot discuss here.

A QUESTION OF ATTITUDE

The essence of yoga is to live our daily life in a yogic poise, or with a yogic attitude. Some vital components of the yogic attitude have been discussed briefly below.

Dealing with the Ego

The ego is the awareness of an individual as a distinct entity. Since this awareness separates the individual from everybody else, it is referred to as the separative ego. In yoga, the separative ego is not considered to be a deep or lasting truth because all creation is a manifestation of the same Divine Consciousness. If this basic truth is grasped, the strangle-hold of the ego is loosened and the individual is overcome by a blissful sense of unity with the rest of this creation. The control, and ultimately the elimination, of the separative ego is an important part of the yogic attitude. With this change of attitude, the person loses his feeling as the doer of his actions. He considers himself merely as an instrument of the Divine. We are often advised 'not to show off' or 'not to think too much of ourselves'. The yogic attitude carries this standard advice to its idealistic culmination. The elimination of the separative ego is the most vital part of the yogic attitude. If this part can be accomplished, the other components outlined below follow as a corollary.

Dealing with Desires

Man is a creature with endless desires. He repeatedly learns that fulfilment of desires does not guarantee perpetual happiness. Once one set of desires is fulfilled, he keeps coming up with new desires and tries frantically to fulfil them. He always seems to be under the illusion that the fulfilment of the latest desire is sure to bring lasting happiness. The reduction, and finally the elimination of desires is also an essential part of the yogic attitude. Many desires are aimed primarily at boosting the ego. Therefore controlling the ego also controls desires. As Sri Aurobindo has pointed out, desires starve in the absence of support from the ego.

Surrender

Surrender requires faith in an all-powerful and all-knowing Being that runs the world in accordance with His designs which are intended to take this world to perfection. Only a person with the ego under control can surrender himself to the will and wisdom of the Supreme.

Equanimity

Surrender enables one to accept victory and defeat, success and failure, happiness and sorrow, with perfect equanimity, and subsequently with the same delight. Such an attitude of equanimity brings lasting inner peace and bliss.

Universal love

Pure love which is extended to all without reservation and without any expectation is a constituent of the yogic attitude. Further, although this love is full of concern, it is devoid of attachment.

Sincerity

In practice, sincerity is the most important virtue. We generally know what to do, but lack the will to do it. Sincerity makes us do the right thing even if it hurts us.

THE HUMAN MACHINE

Using a gadget is great,
But making the machine is greater still.
Inventing the instrument, however,
Needs the greatest skill.

Life is a machine
Invented by the Divine.
Into matter he injects life
To make it a tool divine.

The role of we mortals
Is the simplest of all.
To use the machine
To fulfil His plans big and small.

To do His bidding
Is easier said than done.
The road to His plans
Is blocked by bullies more than one.

The first bully is ego,
A bloated balloon.
Puncture it as you may,
It fills itself soon.

The second bully is desire,
A multiplying tribe.
Oust one, and find two
Begging for a bribe.

Despair not,
For there are friends.

They can facilitate
The journey to His ends.

The first friend is surrender.
Silence your mind,
And you will hear
His voice, clear and kind.

Reason no more,
Do what he says.
Conflict only clouds the vision,
You anyway end up where He takes.

The second friend is merger.
There is after all,
The same divine spark
In beings big and small.

If you are in pain,
I should weep as well.
Your moments of joy
Should make my heart swell.

Merger is easy to preach
But difficult to practise.
That my needs come first,
Is very easy to establish.

To fit into His plans,
There are thus dictums four:
No ego, no desire,
Total surrender, merge more.

YOGIC ATTITUDE IN DAILY LIFE

The yogic attitude might appear to be ideal but too impractical for everyday use. But just knowing about it serves no purpose unless a sincere effort is made to adopt the attitude in daily life. Let us see what it means and how it might be done.

We all do some work, may be for a living or as a hobby. A housewife does plenty of work neither for a living nor as a hobby. How can all these different types of work be done with the same attitude? The yogic attitude to work involves three basic features. First, it is done without a sense of the ego. The person apparently doing the work considers himself to be a mere instrument of the Divine. Second, the work is done without any desire for reward. Third, since the work is done for the Divine, it is given away as an offering to the Divine. Done in this spirit, work brings lasting mental peace. Further, since the work is offered to the Divine, the person tries his best to make the product of the work fit for the Divine. This leads to a level of excellence which may otherwise seem beyond human capabilities. No wonder, the best buildings in the world are places of worship because they are built not for money but for the love of God. The same spirit can be brought also into all our mundane tasks.

In the course of our daily work, we meet several people. A person with a yogic attitude will see all of them as manifestations of the Divine, just like himself. The 'me vs all the rest' divide will fade out. It will be replaced by a vision of the One in all. Once that happens, there is no conflict that cannot be resolved. Tension gives way to harmony. The atmosphere in the workplace will be suffused with peace, friendship and love.

Even simple everyday acts such as eating, sleeping and speaking get transformed by the yogic attitude. Before eating we should say to ourselves that the purpose of eating is to sustain the body so that it can serve as an efficient instrument of the Divine. Before sleeping we should pray that the sleep may restore our strength so that we can resume with renewed vigour, the tasks for which we have been chosen by the Divine. Before speaking we should think a while and let only those words escape our mouth which are consistent with the yogic attitude. Just as our thoughts influence our words, words actually uttered also influence our thoughts. For example, expressing anger in words fuels anger, criticising a person increases our hatred for him, and talking of luxury goods increases our desire to possess them. On the other hand, giving expression to genuine appreciation, love or forgiveness fills us with peace and warmth.

THE YOGIC PRACTICES

We have seen that yoga is a long journey towards perfection. Whenever we are faced with a long journey, we try to hasten our pace by using advanced technology. Yoga also has techniques for increasing the pace of our progress. Asanas and pranayama help us achieve physical improvement, while meditation helps us in the mental sphere. We shall discuss briefly a few yogic practices. This discussion is meant to be only an introduction. For actual performance of the practices, much more guidance – preferably person-to-person – is necessary. Furthermore, persons having some ailments such as heart disease, hernia or back pain would require an appropriate selection of practices because some of the asanas may be harmful for them.

Asanas

Asana, literally, means a posture. Asanas may be classified into three groups depending on their primary purpose: relaxation, physical exercise or meditation.

Asanas for relaxation

These asanas provide physical relaxation, and if properly performed, also mental relaxation. *Shavasana* is the principal asana in this category (Fig. 1.3). It is performed at the beginning and end of a session of asanas, and also sandwiched between some other asanas which provide physical exercise. Another common relaxing posture is *makarasana* (Fig. 1.4). Relaxing asanas may be performed at any time during a session as and when the body becomes tired. They appear simple, but doing them correctly needs practice and patience.

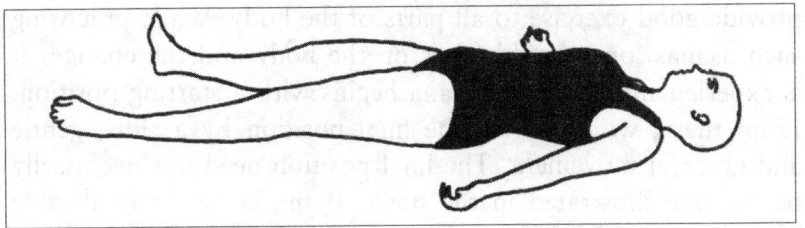

SHAVASANA (The cadaveric posture)

Fig. 1.3. *Shavasana, a posture for relaxation. One should lie down with feet apart, hands away from the body, palms facing upwards, with the eyes closed, and breathe slowly and deeply. As the air goes in, the abdomen goes up, and as the air is breathed out, the abdomen comes down. The whole body should be completely relaxed and the mind should be at peace.*

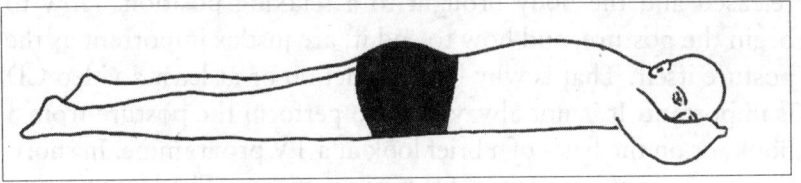

MAKARASANA (The crocodile posture)

Fig. 1.4. *Makarasana, a posture particularly suitable for relaxation between asanas which are performed with the belly touching the ground, such as bhujangasana and dhanurasana.*

Shavasana relaxes the body because all the muscles of the body are relaxed completely through voluntary effort. It also relaxes the mind through slow, deep and conscious breathing, and autosuggestion. *Shavasana* is an extremely useful asana, specially for busy people who are constantly under stress.

Asanas for physical exercise

These asanas are the best known part of yoga. A sequence of 10-15 asanas which would take 30-45 minutes to perform can provide good exercise to all parts of the body. While practising such asanas, one should focus on the body and the changes it is experiencing. A typical asana begins with a starting position. From there, we go on to the final position by a slow, gentle and graceful movement. The final position need not necessarily be the one illustrated in the book. If the body is not flexible enough, it may be difficult. In that case, the right thing to do is to perform the maximum movement in the right direction that can be performed comfortably. As the flexibility of the body improves, it will be possible to get closer to the perfect posture. After reaching the final position – that is, the position which is final for the individual – the posture should be maintained for 5-30 seconds, depending on the capacity of the individual, and the time available. The final position involves intense stretching, but it should be an enjoyable stretch. After that, the posture is released and the body brought to a relaxing position. How to begin the posture, and how to end it, are just as important as the posture itself. That is why live instruction or at least a video CD is important. It is not always safe to perform the posture from a book, or on the basis of a brief look at a TV programme. In short, the sequence of an asana is: Starting position→Final position→Hold→Relaxing posture. After brief relaxation, we perform the counter-pose.[1] That is why, the sequence of asanas also has some importance. If a change is made, at least the pairing of a pose and its counter-pose should not be disturbed.

Several studies have shown the superiority of asanas to ordinary physical exercises in terms of their physical benefits, and even more their psychological benefits and therapeutic effects. Therefore it is natural to a sk how these asanas are different from other physical exercises. The special features of asanas are:

1. The movements are slow, gentle and graceful.
2. Every pose is followed by a counter-pose.

---

[1] If a posture involves bending forward, its counter-pose is a posture which involves bending backward.

YOGA: THE FINEST LIFESTYLE EVER DEVISED 15

3. Stretching alternates with relaxation.
4. The session of asanas begins with relaxation, ends with relaxation, and is interspersed with relaxation.[2]
5. A judiciously designed set of 15-20 postures moves virtually every joint, and stretches every ligament of the body.

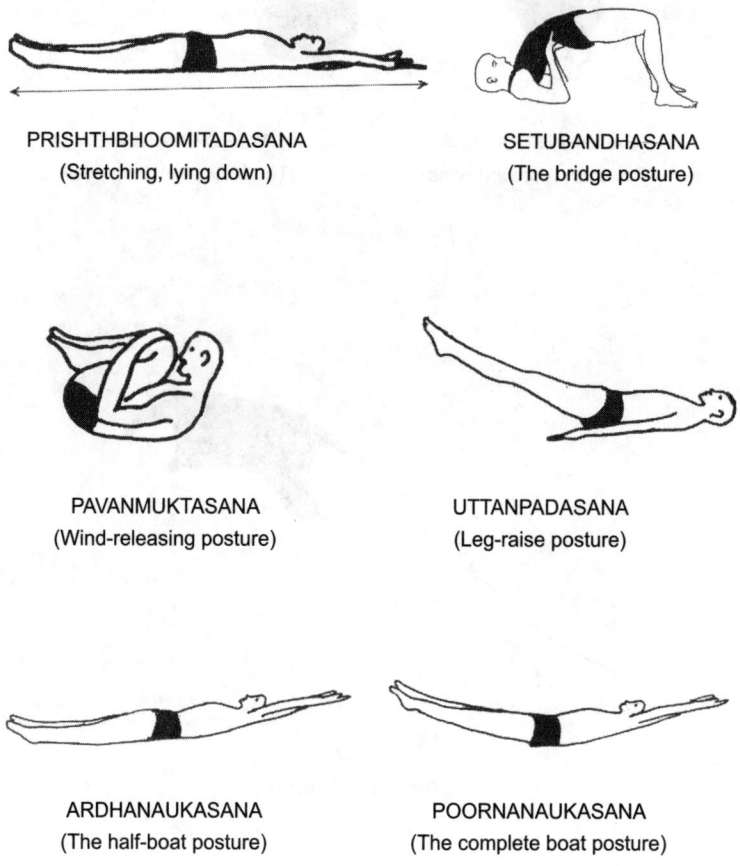

Fig. 1.5. *A set of asanas performed while lying down.*

---

[2] Because of features 2 through 4, at the end of the session, the person is relaxed rather than exhausted.

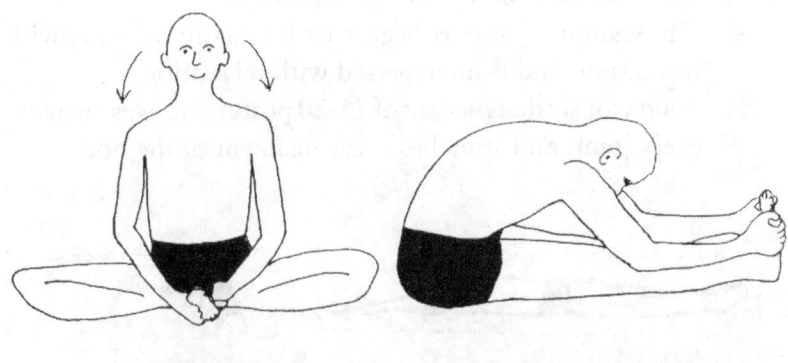

BADDHAKONASANA
(The bound-forward bend)

PASHCHIMATANASANA
(The back stretching posture)

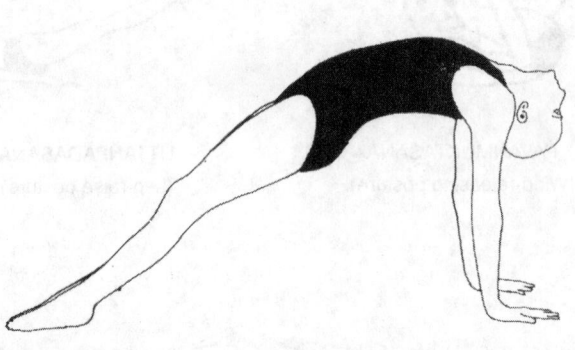

KONASANA
(The inclined plane)

Fig. 1.6. A set of asanas performed sitting up. The arrows in baddhakonasana indicate that after assuming the posture shown, the person bends forward.

Yoga: The Finest Lifestyle Ever Devised 17

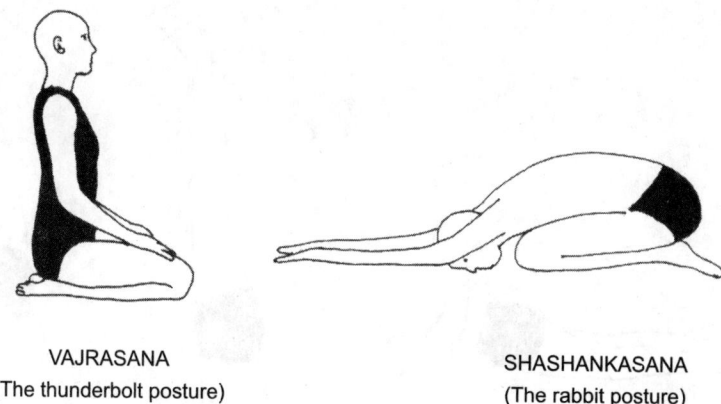

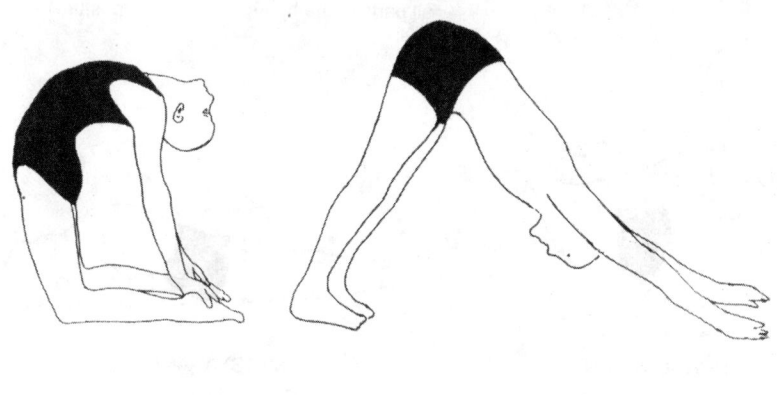

Fig. 1.7. *A set of asanas performed sitting up.*

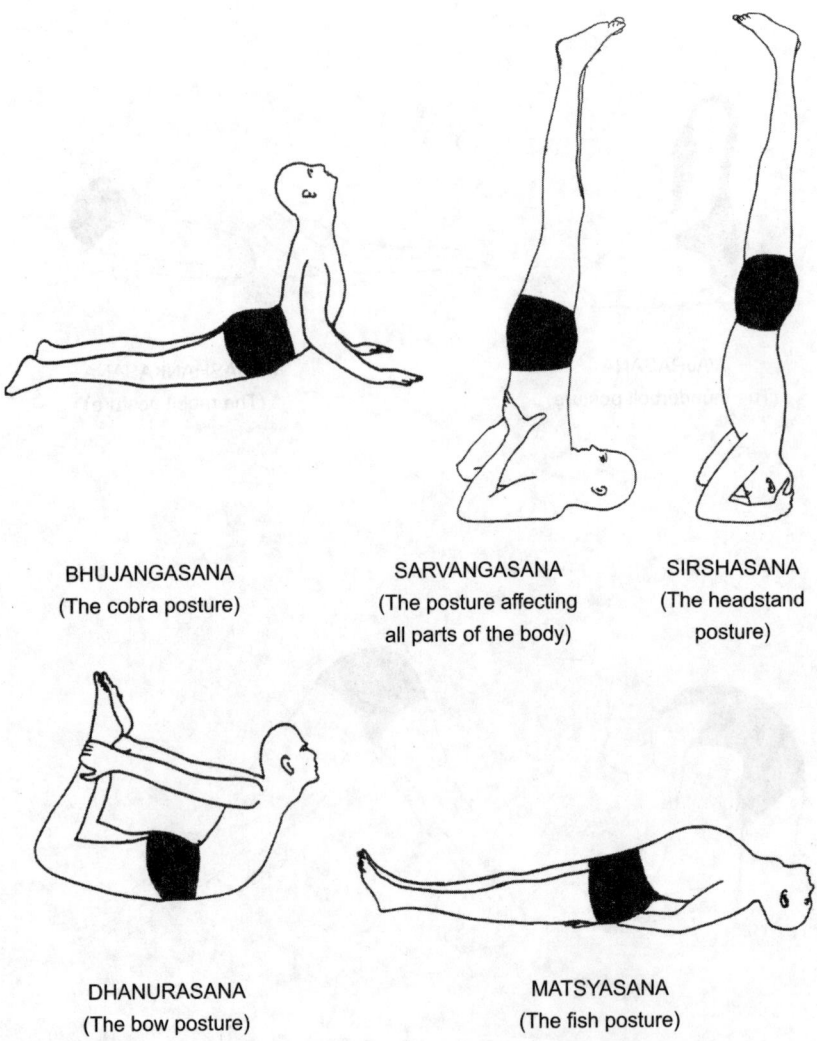

Fig. 1.8. *A set of very popular asanas. Note the similarity between sarvangasana and sirshasana. Both provide similar benefits but sarvangasana is much easier and safer. Sirshasana is a risky posture which should not be attempted by beginners. Sarvangasana is a safe alternative to sirshasana.*

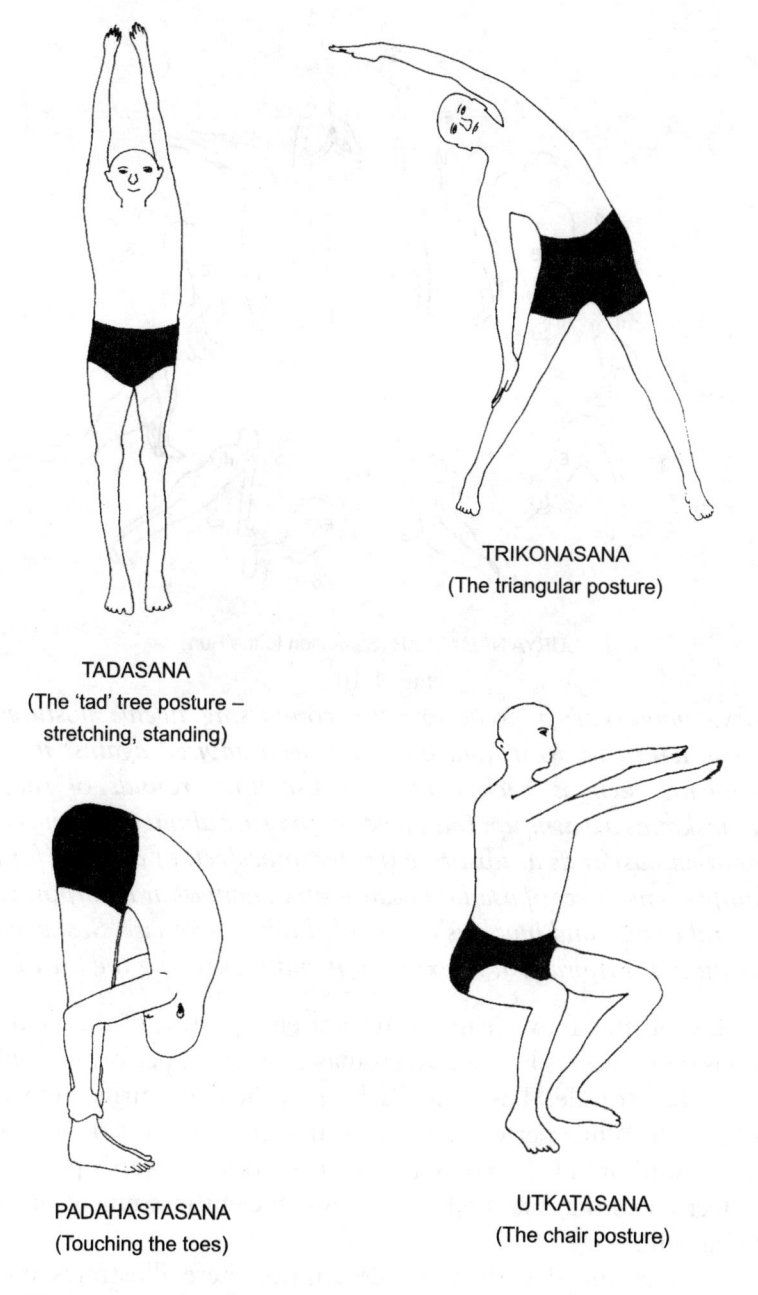

TADASANA
(The 'tad' tree posture – stretching, standing)

TRIKONASANA
(The triangular posture)

PADAHASTASANA
(Touching the toes)

UTKATASANA
(The chair posture)

Fig. 1.9. *A set of asanas performed while standing up.*

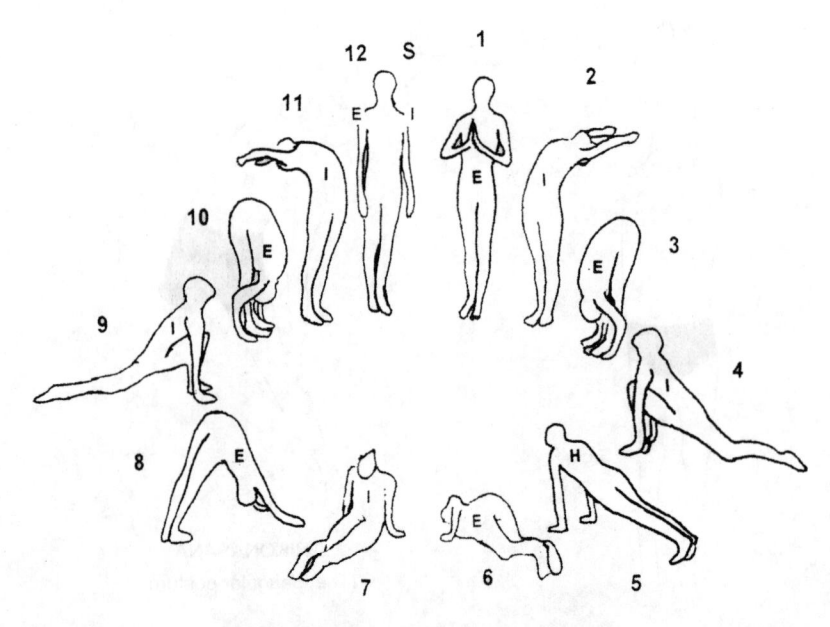

SURYA NAMASKAR (Salutation to the Sun)
Fig. 1.10.

Surya namaskar: a cyclic exercise comprising twelve postures. Those who can do it, and have not been advised against it for problems such as back pain, may use three rounds of surya namaskar as a warm-up. Busy persons may use about six rounds of surya namaskar as a substitute (rather imperfect, of course!) for a comprehensive set of asanas because surya namaskar incorporates several asanas and involves the whole body in exercise. S, starting position; I, inspiration; E, expiration and H, holding the breath.

But all the above features are not enough to call the asanas yogasanas. Asanas become yogasanas only when performed with the right attitude. They should be preceded by purification of behaviour. While performing the asanas, the thoughts occupying the person's mind should be that he is working towards physical perfection so that his body can be an efficient instrument of the divine will.

As mentioned earlier, the description here illustrates only the general principles. It is not adequate for actually performing the asanas. In any case, it is important to bear in mind that the final pose of some asanas may be impossible to achieve for many persons. In such cases it may be harmful to exceed the limits of flexibility of the body. It is enough to make a movement in the right direction with the right attitude although the final pose may not be perfect. Finally, there is only one basic rule for the asanas. They are postures which are steady and comfortable. An unsteady or painful posture is not an asana. Therefore a posture which one finds difficult should not be attempted. Everything cannot be done by everybody in the world.

A reasonable sequence of asanas is given in the accompanying box, and many of the asanas have been illustrated in Figs. 1.5-1.9.

A SEQUENCE OF KEEP FIT ASANAS FOR BEGINNERS
(Duration: about 1 hour)

1.	Warming up	15.	Parvatasana
2.	Shavasana	16.	Makarasana
3.	Prishthbhoomitadasana	17.	Bhujangasana
3a.	*	17a.	Makarasana
4.	Setubandhasana	18.	Dhanurasana
4a.	*	18a.	*
5.	Pavanmuktasana	19.	Sarvangasana
5a.	*	19a.	*
6.	Uttanpadasana	20.	Matsyasana
6a.	*	20a.	*
7.	Ardhanaukasana	21.	Tadasana
8.	Poornanaukasana	22.	Padahastasana
8a.	*	22a.	Tadasana
9.	Baddhakonasana	23.	Trikonasana
10.	Pashchimottanasana	24.	Katichakrasana
11.	Konasana	25.	Utkatasana
11a.	*	25	a *
12.	Vajrasana		
13.	Shashankasana		
14.	Ushtrasana		

* Shavasana
(Courtesy: Sri Aurobindo Ashram – Delhi Branch)
An audiotape providing instructions for these asanas is available from Sri Aurobindo Ashram (Delhi Branch), New Delhi 110 016

PRANAYAMA

Pranayama, literally, means controlling the life force. Since the most visible manifestation of the life force (*prana*) is breathing, pranayama is the term used for a variety of breathing practices. Although we have all been breathing since we were born, most of us do not breathe in the best way. The contrast between the way we generally breathe, and the ideal way to do so has been brought out in Table 1.1.

Table 1.1. THE CONTRAST BETWEEN USUAL BREATHING AND IDEAL BREATHING

Usual breathing	Ideal breathing
Fast	Slow
Shallow	Deep
Predominantly chest breathing (thoracic breathing)	Predominantly abdominal breathing

The reason why slow and deep abdominal breathing is the better way to breathe is that it is more efficient (gets more oxygen in with less effort) and also relaxing. How slow breathing can relax the mind is easy to understand. We have all observed that when we are under stress, we breathe fast; in contrast, when we are relaxed, we breathe slowly. The relationship also works the other way round: when we breathe slowly, we feel relaxed. The simplest form of pranayama (*sahaja* pranayama) basically consists of the right way to breathe, and if we do that for a few minutes everyday, we tend to breathe better throughout the day.

Although, ideally, pranayamas should be done on an empty stomach, and should follow the asanas (and precede meditation), it is often impractical to do all three in the same sitting. In practice, an empty stomach is essential for asanas, but simple pranayamas described below may be practised even two hours after a meal. They may, or may not be immediately preceded by asanas. Thus one may do asanas early in the morning on an empty stomach, but pranayamas at 11 am or 6 pm

Sahaja Pranayama

Sit erect but relaxed. Take a *slow and deep* breath. Make sure that the abdomen moves out as you breathe in. Then breathe out, still more slowly. To achieve the necessary slowness while breathing out, it is helpful if you count mentally from 10 backwards *slowly*, i.e. 10, 9, 8, 7, and so on. Prolong the act of breathing out till you reach 1. Repeat this pattern of breathing a few times. Observe the relaxation you feel at the end of this simple exercise.

Full Yogic Breathing

Sit erect in a comfortable posture. Place one hand on the abdomen and one on the chest. Breathe in slowly. As you breathe in, the abdomen moves out. Continue breathing in, and now the lower and middle part of the chest should expand. Continue breathing in, now using the neck and shoulder muscles. During this stage, the clavicles and shoulders move up. Abdominal, thoracic and clavicular breathing proceed sequentially, but smoothly – without a break. At the end of clavicular breathing, you have inflated your lungs to your utmost capacity. Now start breathing out slowly – in the opposite sequence. First, let the shoulders and clavicles collapse. Then, let the chest deflate. And, finally, let the abdomen move in. The hands on the chest and abdomen help in monitoring the movement of these parts of the body while breathing in and out. It may be helpful to count from 1 to 5 *slowly* while breathing in, and from 10 backwards up to 1 *slowly* while breathing out.

The effect of *sahaja* pranayama and full yogic breathing should spill over to normal breathing throughout the day. It should become natural to breathe a little slower and deeper, and to utilise also abdominal breathing, in addition to thoracic breathing.

Kapalabhati

Kapalabhati, literally, means a shine on the head. It is probably so called because of the feeling of light-headedness at the end of the practice. Normally, we make an effort to breathe in, but breathing out is passive. During *kapalabhati*, breathing out is active, and breathing in is passive. It consists of exhaling forcefully and rapidly using the abdominal muscles, followed by inhaling passively. The rate of breathing in during *kapalabhati* is high. Starting with about 20 strokes per minute, one may speed up the rate as the practice goes on. Towards the end, once again the rate is slowed down before stopping the practice completely. The practice should be limited to about fifteen seconds – continuing it longer might bring on a fainting spell. Experienced practitioners can achieve peak rates of about 120 strokes per minute, and can also continue the practice for longer than fifteen seconds at a stretch without fainting. At the end of the practice, there is no urge to breathe, and in fact breathing might cease for a few seconds. No effort need be made to breathe or to stop breathing – one should just follow what comes naturally and spontaneously.

Although *kapalabhati* does have some benefits, there are many situations in which the harm it may do is greater than its benefits. In these situations, it should not be done. *Kapalabhati* should not be done by those suffering from epilepsy, vertigo, hernia, peptic ulcer, high blood pressure, coronary heart disease, back pain, or neck pain (cervical spondylosis). Further, it should not be done by women during menstruation, or during advanced stages of pregnancy. If in doubt, it is better not to do it. You will not miss much by omitting *kapalabhati*.

Nadi Shuddhi Pranayama

Nadi shuddhi pranayama, or alternate nostril breathing, is called the king of pranayamas. It improves the balance between nostrils, relieves stress, and improves concentration. It never does any harm, and therefore has no contra-indication. It may appear confusing to start with, but becomes quite natural with practice. It helps to remember that the change of nostril should be after each inhalation. In order to block one nostril at a time, the hand is placed in the nasika mudra. Nasika mudra is adopted by folding the two fingers that are just next to the right thumb. The rationale seems to be that in nasika mudra, the distance between the thumb and the ring finger is a little more than the width of the nose. When the right hand in this position is taken towards the nose, the nose fits snugly between the thumb and the ring finger: then, just a little movement of the thumb can block the right nostril, and that of the ring finger can block the left nostril.

Nadi shuddhi pranayama should be done at an even pace, breathing slowly, without making any sound. There is a tendency for the neck to bend forward during the practice, which should be resisted. Keeping so many things in mind, along with flawless alternation of nostrils, needs concentration. It is no wonder then that the practice improves concentration!

Cooling *pranayamas*

Cooling *pranayamas* are performed by breathing in through the mouth and breathing out through the nose. They are so called because of the cooling effect of the cool air entering the airways without warming up in the nose. Although these *pranayamas* are good for high blood pressure, mental stress and nasobronchial allergies, they *should not* be performed if the person has a cold or a sore throat, has sensitive or too many missing teeth, or if the weather is cold or damp.

For breathing in, the mouth should be kept only partially open. The partial opening may be created by rolling the outstretched tongue into a tube (*sitali*), or by folding back the outstretched tongue into the mouth (*sitkari*), or by bringing the edges of the upper and lower teeth in contact (*sadanta*). Any one of the three is enough, and the choice depends on what the person finds the easiest to do. If due to any limitation, the person cannot do the cooling *pranayamas*, he need not worry about it. Not much is missed by omitting any particular yogic technique.

Bhramari

In contrast to the cooling *pranayamas*, during *bhramari*, the person breathes in through the nose, and breathes out through the mouth. While breathing out, the person also chants 'nnn...' loudly, which is a sound resembling that of a female honey bee: hence the name *bhramari*. While chanting, the tongue rolls up to touch the hard palate. The chant produces a soothing resonance in the head. *Bhramari* is said to relieve mental stress, sleeplessness and high blood pressure, and improves the voice. If it is done after taking a deep breath and the chanting continued as long as possible, the duration of the chant is a good indicator of the breath holding time. The regular practice of yogic techniques, specially *pranayamas*, increases the duration of the breath holding time. There is no contra-indication for *bhramari*: anybody may do it.

YOGA FOR HEALTH

The fact that yoga helps promote, preserve and restore health is apparently due to three components of the yogic lifestyle: diet, exercise and mental relaxation.

The yogic diet is usually a simple, fresh, vegetarian diet consumed in just the right amount – neither too much nor too little. Further, the diet is free from items which are not required by the body, such as tea, coffee, alcohol and tobacco. Science now recognises such a diet to be equally suitable for healthy persons as well as for those having any of the diseases of modern civilisation, such as obesity, diabetes mellitus, hypertension and coronary heart disease. In yoga, even more important than the exact items of food consumed and those abstained from, is the attitude to food. To someone doing yoga, food is a necessity, not a sensory pleasure. Therefore, he neither eats out of greed, nor consumes things which are not necessary. He is not preoccupied with food. He consecrates the food with a prayer and then eats it slowly. The inner attitude to food is more important than ritual fasting or symbolic abstinence from certain foods. To paraphrase Sri Aurobindo, without inner renunciation, outer renunciation is of no use. With inner renunciation, outer renunciation is not necessary, although it automatically follows.

The yogic exercises are usually in the form of asanas. But, as discussed earlier, asanas become yogasanas only when performed with the right attitude – one which regards physical perfection to be only a component of overall perfection of the entire being. Performed with this attitude, even a walk can acquire a yogic character.

Yoga generally also involves concentrated efforts at mental relaxation such as meditation. But even more important than these concentrated exercises is the day-long attitude to events and people. Yoga inculcates an all-loving, all-accepting, non-judgmental attitude to life. This attitude is more than mere philosophical indifference. It is an attitude of positive joy and delight, irrespective of external circumstances, because all circumstances are considered a gift from the Almighty, to whose will and wisdom the sadhak has surrendered. The mental peace that this attitude brings has far-reaching implications. The favourable effect of mental relaxation on the heart, stomach, intestines and other organs is well known. Recent scientific studies have shown that one's mental status has a significant impact on the immune status. Mental stress impairs immunity, whereas positive emotions act as immuno-enhancers. Immunity protects the body not only against infections but also against cancer. Thus mental relaxation itself would tend to prevent and alleviate several diseases. Hence yoga, which has an all-pervasive relaxing effect, brings about a remarkable improvement in health which goes beyond the physical effects of exercise and diet.

YOGA AND HAPPINESS

We all wish to be healthy; but even more than that, we wish to be happy. Further, being healthy and happy are only partly related. Doctors sometimes have patients with serious illnesses who are surprisingly cheerful and happy, and even more frequently they have patients with only a minor or imaginary illness who are miserable. In short, happiness does not entirely depend on being healthy. It does not depend on our circumstances but on our attitude to the circumstances. Yoga changes our attitude in a variety of ways to promote happiness in all circumstances. By controlling the ego, we are able to control self-absorption. Extending our love to all further helps in reducing our obsession with ourselves. By controlling our desires, we are not tortured by the anxiety to acquire more and more and by controlling our senses, we are able to exercise a healthy restraint on pursuit of sensory pleasures. By surrendering to the will and wisdom of the Divine, we are able to take delight in whatever comes our way. With virtually all sources of unhappiness thus taken care of, yoga can lead to perpetual calm and delight.

Thus yoga promotes health but cannot guarantee perpetual good health. Even great yogis fall ill, sometimes seriously ill, and they definitely die one day. However, yoga, if followed perfectly, guarantees everlasting peace and joy. Further, the effects of yoga are not confined to the individual. Because of the attitude of the *sadhak* to those around him, the effects of yoga extend to society as a whole.

Frequently Asked Questions

1. *Who is fit to do yoga?*

   Everyone. The path of yoga is open to all. Anyone who feels a call to it should embark on it in all sincerity.

2. *Which type of yoga is easy?*

   None. The sincere pursuit of yoga is an uphill and apparently never-ending quest. Yoga is not easy, but it is enjoyable.

3. *If the whole lifetime may not be sufficient to reach perfection (siddhi), why start doing yoga at all?*

   Fortunately the outcome of yoga is not an all or none phenomenon. Every bit of progress brings commensurate inner peace and joy. The graded nature of the process makes it easy to adopt the dictum, enjoy the journey and forget about the destination.

4. *What is the minimum time required for yoga every day?*

   This is a common question which should not be asked. The question reflects popular misconceptions about yoga. Yoga is not a part time activity. It should influence and ennoble every activity of the day.

5. *Is it incorrect to start asanas before achieving perfection in yama and niyama?*

   No, that would effectively exclude most of us from the practice of asanas. While perfection in *yama* and *niyama* is not a pre-requisite, a conscious effort to enforce them in daily life is highly desirable before starting on asanas.

6. *What time of the day is best for asanas?*

   The best time for asanas is early morning, on an empty stomach, after emptying the bowels. If that is inconvenient, the asanas should be performed more than four hours after the previous meal. For example, if lunch is over at 2 pm, asanas may be performed after 6 pm However, a gap of only half an hour is enough after drinking a liquid. For example, those who must have a cup of tea soon after waking up in the morning may do the asanas thirty minutes after a cup of tea.

7. *How can I find enough time for yogic practices in a busy routine?*

   It is basically a question of will power. One can always find one hour in a day for something which one likes, and which is important. If you are able to continue the practice for a few weeks, you will find that you will start liking it, and will feel as if you are missing something if you do not continue. I find it strange that some people find it easier to do the yogic practices if they pay for classes where they practise the postures in a group for a fixed period at a fixed time everyday. The time taken to travel for the classes is more than the time it would take to do the yogic practices at home. Further, at home, there is some flexibility possible from day to day in terms of when and for how long you wish to practise.

8. *Which practices should I do if I have very limited time, say only about half an hour a day?*

   Here are some of the ways to solve this problem:
   a. If you are young and healthy, you may do a few loosening and breathing exercises as a warm up, about six rounds of *surya namaskar* (Fig. 1.10), and end with about ten minutes of *shavasana*.
   b. If *surya namaskar* is too tough for you, after warming up, you may do the lying down postures one day, and sitting and standing postures the next. You may continue the alternation throughout the week.

   Two things which should not be done even when time is short are:
   a. Do not disturb the pairs of poses and counter-poses. Either do both members of the pair, or omit both.
   b. Do not neglect relaxing asanas such as *shavasana* and *makarasana* at appropriate points.

9. *What should one wear while practising asanas?*

   Any loose and comfortable dress is satisfactory. The dress should not reduce the flexibility of the body. Cotton is better than synthetic fabrics because it lets the sweat evaporate.

10. *Can shirshasana be dangerous?*

    Yes, *shirshasana* is potentially dangerous because it may twist the neck. It is an asana only for experts. Others can derive the benefits of *shirshasana* from the much simpler and safer *sarvangasana*.

11. *What type of diet is suitable for practising yoga?*

    Yogic diet is not a rigid diet. A simple but wholesome vegetarian diet, free from stimulants, is considered the best. However, along with several other desires, the desire for rich food is also likely to disappear gradually as one practises yoga. It is better to change the diet gradually rather than impose a drastic change abruptly.

For Further Reading

1. Iyengar BKS, *Light on Yoga*. New Delhi: HarperCollins, 1966.
2. Nagarathna R, Nagendra HR, *Integrated Approach of Yoga Therapy for Positive Health*. Bangalore: Swami Vivekananda Yoga Prakashana, 2nd Edition, 2004.
3. Pandit MP, *Yoga for the Modern Man*. Pondicherry: Dipti Publications, 1977.
4. Sri Aurobindo, *The Synthesis of Yoga*. Pondicherry: Sri Aurobindo Ashram, 4th Edition, 1970.
5. Sri Aurobindo, *The Integral Yoga. Sri Aurobindo's Teaching and Method of Practice*. Pondicherry: Sri Aurobindo Ashram, 1993.
6. Swami Vivekananda, *Raja-Yoga or Conquering the Internal Nature*. Calcutta: Advaita Ashrama, 22nd Impression, 1995.
7. *The Hathayogapradipika of Svatmarama*. Madras: The Adyar Library and Research Centre, 1972.
8. *Health and Healing in Yoga. Selections from the Mother*. Pondicherry: Sri Aurobindo Ashram, 1979.

2

Demystifying Meditation

*In moments when the inner lamps are lit
And the life's cherished guests are left outside,
Our Spirit sits alone and speaks to its gulfs.*

SRI AUROBINDO

In yoga, meditation has a deep significance. By quieting down the usual surface activity of the mind, meditation allows a better view of the deeper layers of consciousness. There are several systems and techniques of meditation, but they all incorporate some strategy for soothing the mind. Although Patanjali's yoga sutras are among the oldest of the treatises on yoga, they include just about every strategy that has ever been thought of for settling down the turbulence of the mind. Therefore this chapter will be based on these yoga sutras. Patanjali's yoga (also known as raja yoga) describes yoga as an eight-limbed discipline, and is therefore also called *ashtanga* yoga. As discussed in Chapter 1, the first two limbs, *yama* and *niyama*, are essentially dos and don'ts for moral purification. What the sequence signifies is that only after a beginning has been made with becoming a better person is it proper to practise specialised techniques such as meditation. The third limb is asana, and that is what the technique of meditation begins with.

ASANA

Meditation begins with a suitable posture, or asana. Three asanas are generally considered suitable for meditation: *padmasana*, *sukhasana* and *vajrasana* (Fig. 2.1). During *padmasana* or *sukhasana*, the hands may be placed in one of the three positions illustrated in Fig. 2.2. The rationale behind the posture is that the body should be stable and comfortable. If it is difficult to sit in any of the three postures due, for example, to pain in the knees, one may sit on a chair and meditate. If a back support is required, it should be provided. However, the back and neck should be erect, and in one straight line. The rationale for the erect back is that there is less pressure on the lower back when the back is erect than when we slouch forward. Therefore, we can sit for quite a long time without any discomfort with the back erect. The back and neck should be erect, but not tense. It is possible to sit erect and be relaxed. After sitting erect, make a voluntary effort to relax the body. One may start with relaxing the head and neck, and move down part by part to the feet. When the whole body is relaxed, it should feel light and comfortable. It may be easier to relax if the breathing is also slowed down.

It may be asked if one may meditate lying down, since that is the most stable and comfortable posture. The answer is both no and yes: no, because in the lying down posture, we are likely to fall asleep. The answer is also yes because if we wish to meditate at bedtime, falling asleep is not a problem – for that is what we want anyway. And, to fall asleep while meditating, is one of the best ways of falling asleep (Chapter 6).

Most people like to meditate with the eyes closed. However, in some systems of meditation the eyes are kept open, but the visual stimulus is made monotonous by fixing the gaze on some bright spot at the eye level, or on a patch of the floor about a metre in front of the person. The basic idea is to avoid getting distracted by what one is seeing.

PADMASANA
(The lotus posture)

SUKHASANA
(The comfortable posture)

VAJRASANA
(The thunderbolt posture)

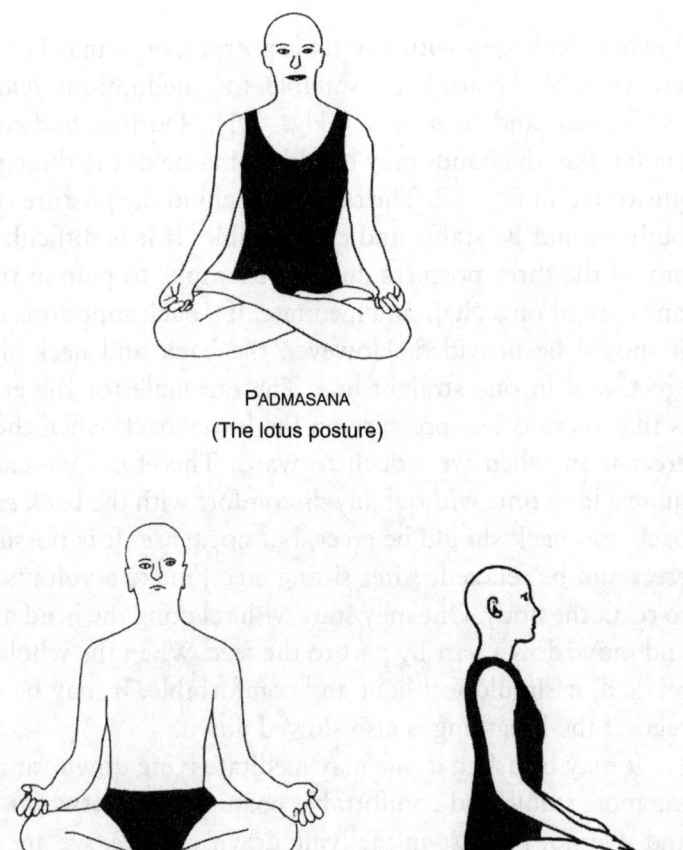

Fig. 2.1. *Asanas suitable for meditation*

Duration, time and place

It is generally recommended that one should meditate for twenty minutes. 'Twenty minutes' is not sacrosanct. In the beginning, twenty minutes may seem too long, and one might make it

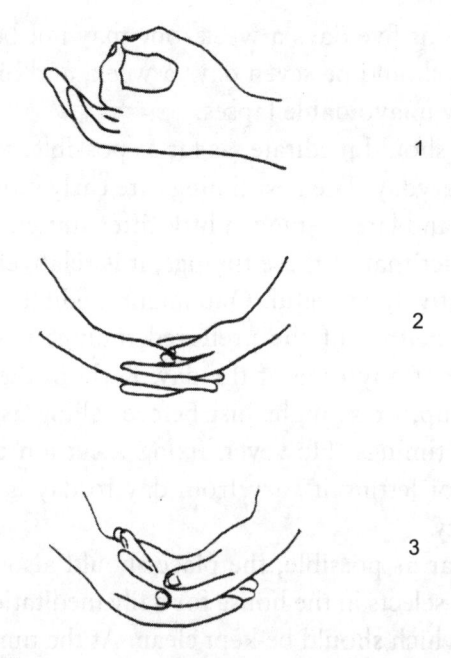

Fig. 2.2. *Three alternative hand positions during meditation:*
1. *Chin mudra*
2. *Interlocked fingers*
3. *One hand cupping the other (Anjali mudra)*

shorter. Later on, one might start enjoying meditating, and might like to go on even beyond twenty minutes. On some days, one might not be able to spare twenty minutes for meditation – in that case, it is much better to meditate for a shorter period than to skip it altogether. One thing which should never be done is to set an alarm for twenty minutes, and as soon as the alarm goes off, we get up with a jerk. Meditation is a peaceful process – one should enter it peacefully, and come out of it peacefully. Coming out of meditation should be a slow, spontaneous and gentle process – meditating for a few minutes longer or less does not really matter. Regularity is far more important than the duration. One cannot compensate for irregularity by meditating longer over the weekend. Regularity means at least five days a week. If one aims at five days a week, one may not be able to stick to it. The aim should be seven days a week, and one may be prepared for a few unavoidable lapses.

One should meditate, as far as possible, at the same time and place everyday. The best timings are early morning, a little before sunrise, and late evening, a little after sunset. The choice depends on the fact that at these timings, it is relatively quiet, and we are also relatively peaceful. One might meditate twice a day, or just once. If neither of the preferred timings is suitable, one might meditate at any time of the day. Early in the morning just after waking up, or at night just before falling asleep, are two other suitable timings. However, fixing a certain time for meditation instead of letting it vary from day to day is helpful in ensuring regularity.

As far as possible, the place should also be fixed. The place that one selects in the house for daily meditation should be a quiet corner which should be kept clean. At the time of meditation, the light should be dimmed and the temperature of the room should be neither too warm nor too cold. The place might be made more conducive to quiet and peace by having a few neutral objects, such as flowers or incense sticks (*agarbatis*); and if one likes, also the pictures of anything or anyone that symbolises the sacred. Settling down at such a place everyday at the same time associates the action with peace, and hence, by itself generates peace.

PRANAYAMA

Having assumed a steady and comfortable posture with the body relaxed and the eyes closed in a comfortable environment, the next step is to attend to the breathing. The rate of breathing is closely related to the state of the mind. It is a common observation that when we are angry, we breathe fast; when we are at peace, we breathe slowly. The relationship holds the other way round also: if we breathe slowly, we feel relaxed. Normally we breathe about fifteen times a minute. During meditation, breathing should be brought down to about five times a minute, that is, just about one-third the normal rate of breathing. In addition, pay attention to the process of breathing. Breathing out should take a little longer than breathing in; and with each inhalation, the abdomen should move out; and with each exhalation, the abdomen should move in. Further, observe that when you breathe in, cool air goes through the nostrils towards the lungs; and when you breathe out, warm air moves from the lungs towards the throat. Do not try to regulate the depth of breathing. At the beginning of the meditation, breathing will be a little deeper than normal, but towards the end of meditation, breathing may be slow and shallow. Let the depth be regulated automatically by the oxygen requirements of the body. You would observe that slow and conscious breathing would itself make you feel very peaceful And some systems of meditation more or less stop there. However, Patanjali knew that the mind would always discover something trivial to engage in. Therefore, he has placed after *pranayama* another step called *pratyahara*.

PRATYAHARA

Pratyahara, in practice, means sensory withdrawal. Several sensory inputs have been taken care of already. The body is stable and comfortable. The eyes are closed: so, we cannot be distracted by what we see. The surroundings are neither too cold nor too warm. However, there is one major sensory input, which still needs to be taken care of. We can still hear the sounds around us. In fact, after you have settled in a meditative posture and have started breathing slowly and consciously, you will start hearing various sounds, such as the sound of the fan in the room, the chirping of birds, horns of vehicles, etc. These sounds might annoy you, or you might think that probably you do not know how to meditate. However, no such reaction is called for – if you do hear such sounds, you should congratulate yourself. The reason why you are hearing these sounds is that you have been so successful in curbing the usual traffic of thoughts that these sounds, which are there in the background all the time but remain unnoticed, become prominent. In short, it is an unmasking effect. Normally, the background noises are masked, or hidden, by the heavy traffic of thoughts. The sounds are there, but we do not notice them. We do not notice them because we do not pay any attention to them – we have far too many thoughts to attend to. Now that all those thoughts have been silenced, the background sounds become conspicuous. Therefore, hearing such sounds is an indication that the meditation is proceeding well. Now all we have to do is to silence these sounds too. For this, a struggle does not help. Just as the best way to still the surface of a pond is to leave it alone, in the same way, these sounds have to be left alone. Pay no attention to the meaning, source or significance of the sounds. If the sounds are ignored, they tend to fade away. That is how we can withdraw from all sensory inputs and achieve *pratyahara*. *Pratyahara*, literally, means 'bringing together' or 'gathering towards'. The mind is normally very restless. It is always crowded with thoughts. Most of these thoughts relate to objects as perceived by the senses. By minimising and ignoring sensory input, the density of thoughts can be reduced. As the density of thoughts decreases, they can be given a certain direction. That is what is meant by 'bringing the thoughts together' or 'gathering them towards' a desired point. Concentrating the thoughts on a point is called *dharana*, which is the next step.

DHARANA

Dharana involves concentration. Let us examine the importance of this step in meditation.

What to concentrate on?

We have already talked about concentrating on the breath. But that is generally not enough to make the mind quiet. Silence is facilitated if we concentrate with all parts of the being. Concentrating on the breath is primarily bodily concentration. If we add a sound, the concentration becomes mental. If the sound is meaningful, the intellect is involved. If the sound has an emotional significance for us, the mind is involved. If the sound is both meaningful and emotionally significant, the head and the heart are both engaged in the concentration. That is why, it is suggested that one should concentrate on either the name of the guru, avatar, god or goddess to whom one is devoted, or a mantra which signifies the sacred to the person who is meditating. Besides the breath and the sound, a material object (eg a flower or a picture), a flame, a thought, an idea, or a part of the body are also suitable for concentrating on. Although there is no limit to what one may concentrate on, the breath and a sound are among the commonest objects of concentration.

How to concentrate?

The concentration on the breath, at least the slowing of the breath should continue during *dharana*. If a sound is added to the object of concentration, the breathing and the sound should be synchronised so that they form one unit. If it is a short sound, it may be recited while breathing out. If it is a longish sound, it may be split into two – the first part may be recited during inspiration, and the second during expiration. The recitation may be loud or silent, but silent recitation is more conducive to the silence of the mind.

Why concentrate?

Dharana, or concentration, has two roles to play during meditation. First, it gives the mind something to be busy with. In Kerala, there is a festival called Puram during which elephants are taken in a procession through the city. The route of the procession might pass through narrow streets, and some of these streets have shops which sell coconuts. The elephants enjoy picking up a coconut with the trunk and swallowing it up. The mahout does not want this and therefore, right at the outset, he gives the elephant a stick to hold in the trunk. The elephant thinks that it has been given a job to do. It also knows that if it tries to pick up a coconut, the stick will drop. Now it gladly goes through the procession without touching a coconut. The sound that we concentrate on during meditation serves exactly the same function as the stick does for the elephant. Our mind gets a job to do, and is therefore less likely to go astray. However, if that were the only function of *dharana*, a neutral sound, such as 'one' should be as good as any other sound. But a neutral sound does not generate peace and silence as efficiently as a sound which symbolises the Divine. This possibly happens because repeating the sound with each breath gives the person who is meditating the assurance that to his own feeble efforts has been added the force of the omnipotent. The association of the force with the sound is strengthened as time goes by, with the result that those who has been meditating for years might experience more or less instant peace as soon as they start their recitation. For this very reason, once a sound has been selected, it should not be changed, at least not changed too often, as it will hamper the development of the association between the force and the sound.

DHYANA

Dhyana actually means meditation. The word *zen* has also been derived from *dhyana*. Although many systems of meditation stop with concentration, Patanjali knew that if a person concentrates on the same object regularly, he might get some thoughts related to the theme of concentration itself. These thoughts, which emanate from the object of concentration, need not be checked. These thoughts constitute *dhyana*. Thus *dhyana* is development and elaboration of the theme of concentration and can assume several forms. For example, if a person is concentrating on his guru's name, he might see the guru's image, start pondering over the guru's teachings, or initiate a dialogue with the guru. These thoughts should be allowed to run on freely, and when they stop, one should return to *dharana*. Thus one may keep going back and forth between *dharana* and *dhyana*. *Dharana* is akin to focusing, and *dhyana* to defocusing. While the repetition during *dharana* is the same everyday, the thoughts or images during *dhyana* need not be. The steps in meditation from *pratyahara* through *dhyana* have been shown diagrammatically in Fig. 2.3.

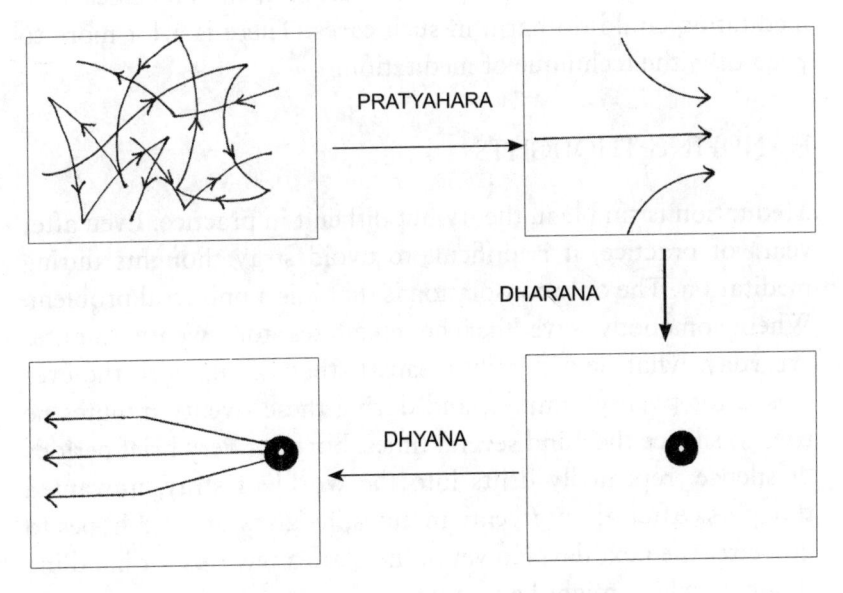

Fig. 2.3. *Progressive steps in meditation.*

SAMADHI

The last limb of Patanjali's yoga is *samadhi*. *Samadhi* is not a part of the process of meditation: it is the product of meditation. *Samadhi* is not something 'to be done'; it is something 'that happens'. Since *samadhi* is an experience, it cannot be described adequately. It is an experience in which the distinction between the subject (who is meditating) and the object (of his meditation) disappears. There is often an intense desire among those who meditate to experience *samadhi*. The desire delays the experience. In fact, absence of this desire is itself a sort of *samadhi*. The aspiration for progress in yoga should be intense and sincere, but not impatient. The effort should be calm and steady, not restless and driven by desire. Anxiety and impatience may sometimes lead to experiences which might be mistaken for *samadhi*. These experiences may at best be glimpses of the state of *samadhi*, and could even be hallucinations. These hallucinations could worsen the condition of people with certain mental illnesses. And meditating could do harm in such cases. There is a lot more to yoga than the technique of meditation.

HANDLING THOUGHTS

Meditation is simple in theory but difficult in practice. Even after years of practice, it is difficult to avoid stray thoughts during meditation. The only consolation is that it is a universal problem. When somebody says that he meditates for twenty minutes everyday, what he generally means is that he sits with the eyes closed for twenty minutes, and during these twenty minutes he tries to silence the mind several times, but after very brief periods of silence, repeatedly drifts into the world of stray, unwanted thoughts. After about twenty minutes, he gives up, and hopes to do better the next day. However, there are a few tips for handling thoughts which might be useful.

Ignore

Do not pay any attention or importance to the thought. Adopt, what is called, a spectator (*drashta*), or a witness (*sakshi*) attitude. Here is an analogy: so many letters enter the postbox everyday, and are removed periodically by the postman. The letters include love letters, 'hate letters', and letters full of complaints and appreciation, grievances and gratitude. The postbox is not affected by the contents of the letters. Letters come and go, but the postbox remains the same. Let your mind become like the postbox. The thoughts should come and go, but your mind should remain the same. This technique can be so effective that just moments after you have detached yourself from a thought, it may become impossible to recollect what the thought was. This method of handling thoughts is most effective in case of thoughts which have been going on in the mind for some time. These thoughts enter the mind unawares, and only after they have engaged the mind for some time that the person becomes aware of their being out of place during meditation. Then it does not pay to get disturbed or agitated. The best policy is to just distance yourself from the thought, and let it fade away.

Reject

This is a more active method of handling thoughts. The thought is rejected, actively. This method is suitable only for the thoughts which have been detected right at their inception. If the thought is detected before it enters the mind, it can be stopped at the threshold; it can be nipped in the bud.

Record

When you sit down to meditate, keep a paper and a pencil handy so that a thought may be scribbled. This method is suitable only for thoughts about things to be done. For example, when you sit down to meditate, you might suddenly remember that you must make a phone call immediately after the meditation. Or, a housewife might remember that she must take the curd, and put it in the refrigerator. These thoughts have a tendency to become recurrent. To prevent this, a simple way is to scribble it on paper. The eyes may be closed while writing, but still whatever squiggles are left on the paper will be sufficiently legible to recollect the task that you wanted to record. This simple act prevents recurrence of such thoughts by reassuring us that since the task has been recorded, it will not be forgotten. Thus you may end up creating a short list of 'things to do' during meditation.

Once a thought has been handled by the most appropriate method, one should return to *dharana*, even if the thought had occurred during *dhyana*. It is much easier to return to mechanical repetition of a sound than to *dhyana*. From *dharana*, one may drift into *dhyana*, and after some time, again return to *dharana*. Thus it is quite acceptable and normal to keep going back and forth between the two.

VISUALISATION AND IMAGERY

If the person is interested in using meditation for health-related gains, towards the end of meditation he may spend a few minutes on visualisation. Visualisation may be coupled with *dharana*. Visualisation may be general, for the body as a whole to grow stronger and healthier, or for a particular part that is diseased. If it is general, one may visualise during each inspiration a wave rising up the spine and spreading out in the skull like a funnel. During expiration, one may visualise divine grace being poured into the funnel, travelling down the spine, and leaking out of the spine to spread throughout the body, invigorating the body, and correcting any derangements anywhere in the body. The sound on which you may be concentrating during *dharana* is also recited at least partly during expiration. Most of the sounds chosen for concentration tend to end in an 'm' or 'n', and are humming sounds (eg *om, amen, ameen, shalom*, etc). If you prefer a non-religious sound, *'maa'* is a good choice, and the sound may mean to you the Mother, a goddess, or your mother. Humming sounds produce a vibration, or resonance, in the body, even if the sound is recited silently. Couple this resonance with the wave spreading throughout the body during expiration (Fig. 2.4). If the visualisation is directed towards a specific part of the body, the general principle remains the same. However you may 'direct' the

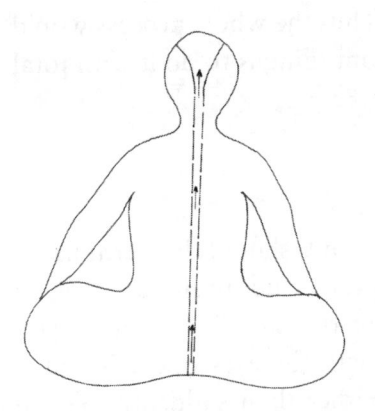

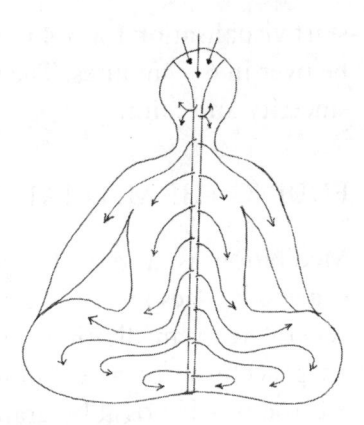

Fig. 2.4. *A suggested image for general well being. During inspiration, visualise a wave rising up the spine, and spreading out into a funnel-like structure when it reaches the head. During expiration, visualise divine grace entering your body through the funnel. Visualise the descending wave charged with divine energy spreading down and radiating throughout the body, creating a healing resonance wherever it goes.*

wave of resonance towards the organ affected. Further, you may visualise healing changes in the organ as the wave travels through the organ. The image of healing changes that you create need not be anatomically correct – in fact, you can give full play to your imagination during the imagery. You will find a few such examples of imagery in Chapters 10, 13 and 14. Feel free to devise your own images for any organ. There is evidence that the approach works. The mind-body relationship is so deep that if you think repeatedly that something is happening to your body, it tends to actually happen. However, do not depend only on imagery for treatment! While using imagery for a specific disease, it is better to do it for 3-4 minutes at a time, 2-3 times a day. The meditation need not last for 20 minutes each time. In a 20-minute meditation, visualisation is restricted to the last 5 minutes or so. When you are just interested in visualisation, you may cut short the earlier steps, and within a minute or two of reaching *dharana*, you may start visualisation for 3-4 minutes. Thus the whole process would be over in 6-7 minutes. The important thing is to do it with total sincerity and faith.

ENDING THE MEDITATION

Meditation is a peaceful process, and should be terminated peacefully. Resolve to keep the peace and positive thoughts generated by meditation throughout the day. Blink yours eyes. Sit peacefully for a few moments with the eyes open. Brighten the room – if possible, gradually rather than suddenly. Get up slowly, holding on to a wall or a door handle for support – taking support is particularly important for the elderly. Walk slowly on your way to resuming your normal activities.

CLOSING THOUGHTS

Unwanted and random thoughts are the commonest and most difficult problem to solve during meditation. The problem needs infinite patience and perseverance. To achieve perfect silence of the mind, even years of practice may not be enough, but with sincere efforts, progress is certain. The aspiration should be intense, but impatience is undesirable. Being in a hurry does not go well with the spirit of meditation. The process of meditation may be summarised as follows:

1. Assume the right posture at a fixed time and place. Close your eyes.
2. Breathe slowly and concentrate on the process of breathing.
3. Try to achieve total sensory withdrawal.
4. Concentrate on a chosen sound, object or idea, and synchronise it with breathing.
5. Let the mind dwell on the object of concentration. Feel free to go back to concentration as and when you like.
6. Terminate the meditation gently when you feel like it.

Frequently Asked Questions

Which are the parts of the body suitable for concentrating upon?

The area in front of the heart, or the point between the eyebrows, is the part of the body most suitable for concentrating on during *dharana*. This concentration can also be synchronised with breathing. When that is done, the part of the body one is concentrating on seems to pulsate rhythmically with each breath.

3
Eating Wisely and Well

Fad diets are bad diets.
SIR STANLEY DAVIDSON

Everyone accepts that there is an intimate relationship between what we eat and our health. Besides what we eat, how much we eat and the attitude with which we eat are equally important. In this chapter, we shall approach the subject of nutrition through nutrients, the chemical constituents of foods. The reason behind starting with nutrients is that it simplifies the subject. To give an analogy, starting with a few basic yarns such as cotton, wool, silk and polyester, we manufacture a wide variety of textiles. Further, by cutting and stitching the cloth in different ways, we make a still wider variety of garments. In the same way, nature has packed a few basic nutrients in different permutations and combinations in a wide variety of foods. Further, by cooking these foods in different ways, we get a still wider variety of recipes.

WHAT IS FOOD MADE UP OF?

Chemically, the chief constituents of all foods are one or more of the following:
1. Carbohydrates

2. Proteins
3. Fats
4. Vitamins
5. Minerals
6. Water
7. Other nutrients

Carbohydrates

Carbohydrates may be called the 'Cinderella' of nutrition. They do most of the work, providing up to 80 per cent of the energy in some diets, and yet are treated as an embarrassing aspect of the Indian diet. We need no longer feel apologetic about the high carbohydrate content of Indian diets. The science of nutrition has travelled full circle, and high-carbohydrate diets can stand on their own merit as among the finest that have ever been devised. However, all carbohydrates are not alike. Broadly speaking, there are two types of carbohydrates: starch and sugar. Starch is a complex carbohydrate, whereas sugar is a form of simple carbohydrate. Complex carbohydrates are preferable to simple carbohydrates for a variety of reasons, which have been summarised below.

1. Starch takes more time and effort on the part of the gut to digest and absorb than sugar. Therefore, the rise in the level of blood sugar is much greater after consuming sugar than after consuming starch, although the amount of carbohydrate in both the meals may be the same. This makes starch much better than sugar for prevention as well as treatment of diabetes (Fig. 3.1).
2. Starch is consumed primarily in the form of grains (cereals and pulses). Grains contain not only starch but protein too, a small but adequate quantity of essential fat, vitamins, minerals and fibre. This makes grains a package deal: they provide all the major nutrients we need in a decent quantity. In contrast,

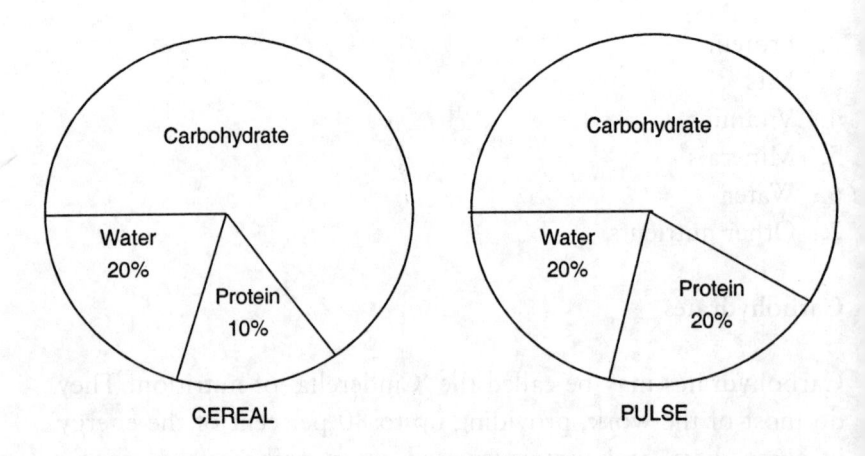

Fig. 3.1. *Approximate composition of a typical cereal and pulse. Note that both have plenty of carbohydrate (starch). Further, cereals also have protein.*

sugar is 100 per cent carbohydrate. Such purity is undesirable in nutrition because we need a variety of nutrients.

3. Starchy foods take time and effort to chew. In contrast, sugar enters the body rather silently. It is present in easy-to-eat foods without making any obvious difference to their weight or volume, and makes them more palatable. The result is that when we eat sweets, we end up overeating. This increases the risk (Chapter 8).

4. Sweets tend to stick between the teeth. Food sticking between the teeth gets fermented by germs in the mouth. Fermentation produces acid. Acid dissolves the enamel of the teeth, producing dental cavities. Therefore we should wash our mouth immediately after a meal. Immediately means at once, because even a few minutes delay significantly increases the risk for cavities.

Besides cereals and pulses, potatoes and bananas are also good sources of starch. One gram of carbohydrate gives four calories of energy to the body.

Proteins

There are a few misconceptions about proteins which need to be clarified. It is sometimes believed that protein is a good nutrient, and therefore the more the better. We should get enough protein, but an excess is unnecessary and could even be harmful. Secondly, it is commonly thought that among vegetarian foods, only pulses (dals) and milk have protein. The fact is that, as in case of carbohydrates, we get most of our protein also from cereals and pulses. Although cereal and pulse proteins individually are of poor quality, a mixture of the protein from the two is good. This is so because cereal and pulse proteins are differently deficient. When the two are combined, the deficiency in cereal protein is made up by pulse protein, and the deficiency in pulse protein is made up by cereal protein. Further, the quantity of protein in a diet, in which staple foods are cereals and pulses, is also adequate. Thus a cereal-pulse mixture can look after our energy needs and also our protein needs – both in terms of quantity as well as quality. Milk and milk products, eggs, and meat are other sources of protein, but cereals and pulses are the major sources of protein in most Indian diets, and that is scientifically satisfactory. One gram of protein gives four calories of energy to the body.

Fats

We get some fat from cereals and pulses, which is sometimes called invisible fat because it is not obvious. Strictly speaking, the invisible fat supplied by cereals and pulses is enough to meet the essential fat requirements of the body. Therefore, theoretically, a zero-oil diet can be suffcient. But most diets also contain some visible fat in the form of oils, butter and ghee. Within reasonable limits, visible fat is well tolerated provided it comes from the right sources. Opinion about what the right sources are has changed dramatically during the last few decades. Based on current scientific knowledge, the best oils are mustard oil and soyabean oil. They may be combined with a small amount of saturated fats such as butter, ghee or palmolein. As a rule of thumb, the visible fat consumption of an adult should be less than one kilogram per month. One gram of fat gives nine calories of energy to the body.

Vitamins and Minerals

Vitamins and minerals do not give energy but are essential for performing many other functions in the body. It is difficult to get enough vitamins and minerals from cereals and pulses and we have to depend on vegetables and fruits. Most of us consume very little of these foods. The current recommendation is that every adult should take about 400 g of vegetables and fruits every day. We need fruits and vegetables not only for vitamins and minerals but also for fibre and phytochemicals. We also get fibre from cereals and pulses, but grain fibre is chemically different from vegetable and fruit fibre, and the two have somewhat distinct and complementary functions.

Water

Water is seldom considered a nutrient. But we need at least a litre of water every day. Come summers, we may need 3-4 litres to compensate for loss through perspiration. Inadequate water intake predisposes one to urinary stones as well as urinary infections.

Other nutrients

Although the six nutrients discussed briefly above are the classic well-established nutrients, several other substances found in plant foods in small quantities (collectively called phytochemicals) may act as antioxidants, immuno-enhancers, hypolipidemic agents, anti-diabetic factors, anti-infective agents and anti-tumour agents. The most common phytochemical is dietary fibre. Fibre is indigestible but has important functions. It prevents constipation, and may also play a role in prevention of diabetes, heart disease, gall bladder stones and cancer of the large intestine. Therefore we should consume plenty of fruits and vegetables to get a good supply of phytochemicals. Since spices are a concentrated source of phytochemicals, a good diet should also have spices in moderation.

Anti-oxidant pills, interestingly, do not confer the same degree of protection as vegetables and fruits. Thus, there is no substitute for natural foods.

A CLOSER LOOK AT DIFFERENT KINDS OF FOOD

Now let us synthesise the above information in terms of the commonly consumed foods.

Cereals

Cereals such as wheat and rice are our staple food. Most cereals contain carbohydrate (about 70 per cent), protein (about 10 per cent) and water (about 20 per cent) (Fig. 3.1). Cereals also contain small but useful quantities of fat and fibre. Please note that cereals do contain protein. In fact, since cereals are our staple food, we get 80 per cent of our protein from cereals. Secondly, unrefined cereals have more dietary fibre as well as more vitamins and minerals than refined cereals. Therefore cereals should be preferably consumed unrefined, i.e. with the husk. Thus brown rice is better than white rice, and atta is better than maida.

Pulses

Pulses (dals) are an important part of our diet. Their composition is similar to that of cereals. Most pulses contain carbohydrates (about 60 per cent), proteins (about 20 per cent) and water (about 20 per cent) (Fig. 3.1). Like cereals, they also have useful quantities of fat and fibre.

We do not depend upon pulses to make our dietary supply of protein adequate. The principal significance of pulses in our diet is that their protein complements the quality of cereal protein. Like cereals, pulses should also be preferably consumed unrefined, i.e. with the husk intact. Thus whole (*sabut*) dals are better than dehusked (*dhuli*) dals.

Vegetables and Fruits

Most of the vegetables and fruits constitute more than 80 per cent water. But the remaining 10-20 per cent provides significant and much-needed quantities of vitamins, minerals, dietary fibre and phytochemicals. Among vegetables, green leafy vegetables are particularly important. Further, as far as possible, vegetables should be consumed raw to avoid cooking losses. From the scientific point of view, there is no difference between vegetables eaten raw and fruits. There is no relationship between the nutritive value of a fruit and its price. Therefore, consuming expensive fruits is not necessary for staying healthy. According to current recommendations, we should consume 400 g of vegetables and fruits every day. Most of us consume far less of these foods than is desirable. Although these foods take time and effort to chew, and are not the most palatable part of the meal, their importance makes it all worthwhile. A simple way to ensure adequate intake of vegetables and fruits is to take five helpings of these everyday. One could include a fruit in the breakfast, and a cooked vegetable and a helping of salad at lunch as well as dinner; that makes five helpings. If each helping is about 100 g, it would ensure an intake of at least 400 g of vegetables and fruits in a day.

Milk

Milk is often referred to as an ideal or complete food. This is not entirely true. While milk has carbohydrate, good protein and fat, it cannot fully meet our requirement of vitamins and minerals. Therefore only children under six months of age can subsist entirely on milk. Some adults cannot digest milk well. They can generally get the benefits of milk from curd. Besides, curd also offers special protection to the intestines, which makes it a very desirable item in the diet. Milk in the diet supplies calcium. Further, in a vegetarian diet, milk is the only source of vitamin B_{12}. For fulfilling both these roles, about 200 ml of milk is quite adequate.

Eggs

Except for the absence of carbohydrates, eggs have almost all other important nutrients. Many adults avoid eggs due to their cholesterol content. One egg has 250 mg of cholesterol. Fortunately, an average Indian diet does not have any other major source of cholesterol, and for healthy adults it is permissible to take up to 300 mg of cholesterol per day. Therefore taking one egg per day still leaves the cholesterol intake of most Indians within the permissible limit. Patients with high blood cholesterol or coronary heart disease should, however, follow their physician's advice.

Fats and oils

They provide only fat, and should be taken, if at all, in proper combinations (as indicated earlier) and in modest amounts. Their intake is not strictly necessary because the minimum quantity of fat essential for the body is available from the usual intake of cereals and pulses.

Spices

Spices are a concentrated source of phytochemicals. Therefore a moderate amount of spices helps in improving the diet. If some spices like red chillies do not suit a person due to acidity or piles, several other spices such as turmeric, methi, garam masala, ginger and garlic may still be consumed.

Meat

Meat is essentially a source of good quality protein (about 20 per cent) and water (about 80 per cent). Some meats also have considerable quantity of saturated fat. No meat contains any dietary fibre. Further, just as several protective factors have come to light in plant foods, some factors predisposing to cancer have been found to be associated with meat. Because of all these reasons, diets containing large amounts of meat are no longer considered healthy. Rather, there is a strong opinion favouring vegetarian diets.

A BALANCED DIET

Balance is a basic principle of life and this applies to diet as well. A balanced diet contains all the necessary nutrients in just the right amount. As discussed above, a combination of cereals and pulses can take care of our energy and protein needs, and also provide us some fibre, essential fats, vitamins and minerals, specially if the grains are not highly refined. To further supplement fibre, vitamin and mineral intake, vegetables and fruits are essential. Finally, to meet calcium and vitamin B_{12} requirements, milk is invaluable. Judiciously selected fats and oils, in moderation, are also acceptable, although not essential. Spices, in moderation, are also desirable for their content of a large variety of protective factors. Thus in the context of Indian diets, a balanced diet is a predominantly vegetarian diet in which the staple foods are cereals and pulses, preferably unrefined; which has about 400 g of vegetables (preferably the green leafy ones) and fruits, at least part of the vegetables being uncooked; which has about 200 ml of milk or milk products (preferably curd); which has a moderate amount of judiciously chosen fat; and which also has a moderate amount of spices. This is a diet which is healthy for a person who is fit, and also good for a person having diabetes or a heart disease (also see Chapters 10 and 11). A basic principle of balanced diets is that they contain a variety of foods. Keeping this basic principle in mind, if one enlarges the variety, firstly it makes the diet more palatable, and secondly it ensures that not only well established but also minor and poorly understood nutrients will be present in the diet in adequate amount.

ASSESSING YOUR OWN DIET

You may like to assess your own diet. Assessment has two aspects – qualitative and quantitative, and both are important. Qualitatively, your diet should answer 'yes' to the following questions:

1. Does it have a mixture of cereals and pulses as the main component?
2. Does it provide more than 400 g of vegetables and fruits everyday?
3. Does it have the right type of oil(s) in moderation?
4. Are the cereals and pulses in the diet consumed along with the husk?

Quantitatively, you should know your energy requirements, and the diet should supply it. You may be able to get a rough idea of your energy requirements from Table 1. Next, you should know your energy intake. A rough idea of your energy intake may be had from Table 2.

Table 1. RECOMMENDED ENERGY INTAKE FOR INDIAN ADULTS*

	Body weight (kg)	Physical Activity	Energy intake per day (Calories)
Men	60	Mild	2425
		Moderate	2875
		Heavy	3800
Women	50	Mild	1875
		Moderate	2225
		Heavy	2925

*As recommended by the Indian Council of Medical Research

Table 2. APPROXIMATE ENERGY CONTENT OF COMMON FOOD ITEMS

Recipe	Energy (Calories)
Chapatti (one)	100
Paratha (one)	275
Dosa, sada (one)	130
Idli (one)	100
Dal (one katori)	100
Banana (one, medium-sized)	150
Apple (one, medium-sized)	70
Orange (one, medium-sized)	60
Milk (one glass, with sugar)	180
Egg (one)	80
Burfi (one piece)	100
Gulab jamun (one)	100
Rasgulla (one)	100
Ice cream (100 ml)	100
Samosa (one, medium-sized)	250
Vada (one, medium-sized)	200
Sugar (one teaspoonful)	20

Next, you can check whether your energy requirement matches well with your energy intake. Note that the tables which have been provided are very incomplete and highly condensed, and therefore quite inaccurate. Therefore it would not be proper to draw any definite conclusions from them. Further, no such tables in the world, no matter how comprehensive, can tell you whether you are eating exactly as much as you need! If that is so, you may wonder what is the use of going through the cumbersome process. The use is that you may enjoy the exercise. However, if you don't, there is a simpler and more pragmatic way of knowing whether you are eating right quantitatively. If your body weight is constant, you are eating right; if you are gaining weight, you are probably eating too much; if you are losing weight, it may be because you are not eating enough (but it may be because of a disease, for which medical advice is necessary). If you are gaining weight and are sedentary, it will be better to increase your physical activity instead of reducing your food intake.

Frequently Asked Questions

1. *What are the recent advances in methods of losing weight?*

    This is one area where one can say that 'new is not good, and good is not new'. The really good approaches are time-honoured and well-known: eat less and exercise more (for more details, see Chapter 8).

2. *Why is it said that one should eat a variety of foods?*

    This is basically a sound principle in nutrition. No single food can meet all our needs. But the nutrients missing in one food can easily be obtained from another. Therefore a variety of foods generally ensures adequate supply of all nutrients. However, one should keep two things in mind. First, the variety should be judiciously chosen – any indiscriminate assembly of foods will not ensure adequate nutrition. Secondly, variety beyond a point may be unnecessary, and may promote overeating, and consequently overweight.

3. *Is non-vegetarian food essential for good health?*

    No, it is just as possible to be healthy and strong on a vegetarian diet as on a non-vegetarian one. On the contrary, several anti-infective, anti-cancer and anti-oxidant chemicals are found only in plant foods, and some undesirable cancer-inducing substances are found in animal foods.

4. *Is liking for certain foods a good guide for our nutritional needs?*

    In general, it is a rather poor guide. Those who lose more salt in urine due to a hormonal deficiency do like salt. But apart from this there is no other well-established relationship between likes and bodily needs. Rather, most foods that most people love are harmful in some way. This applies to highly refined food, fried food, foods which have undergone elaborate cooking and processing, and sweets. Therefore when people are advised to regulate their diet in the interest of health, they find the change hard but may comply half-heartedly accepting it as a necessary evil. The yogic attitude makes it easier to have food that is good for the body, and to take it happily. In short, what is *shreyas* (good) also becomes *preyas* (pleasant).

5. *Does food influence our thoughts and personality?*

Not always, but the possibility exists. It is easy to accept that our thoughts influence our actions. For example, the yogic attitude affects what we eat. The converse is also true: our actions can also influence our thoughts. Eating a vegetarian diet with the conscious objective of kindness to animals is thus likely to make us more compassionate.

6. *What is dietary fibre, and why is it required?*

Fibre is a group of substances, mostly carbohydrates, present only in plant foods, which are not digested by the juices available in the stomach or intestines. Being indigestible, these substances reach the large intestine as such. Further, these substances hold water. Therefore fibre increases the bulk of the residue in the large intestine and makes the residue soft. Both these actions help in preventing constipation. Constipation is not just an inconvenience: it is also the mother of serious problems like varicose veins, piles and hernia. Further, fibre also slows down the digestion of other nutrients, thereby reducing the rise in blood glucose following a meal. Therefore it helps in the prevention and treatment of diabetes. Through some other subtle local and metabolic effects, fibre is also known to help in the prevention of heart disease and cancer of the large intestine.

7. *How can we get dietary fibre?*

   We can get it from unrefined grains (cereals and pulses) as well as vegetables and fruits. We should get it from both these sources because the predominant types of fibre in these are different, and have different types of physiological effects.

8. *What is wrong with sugar?*

   There is a lot that is wrong with sugar, although only indirectly. Sugar is 100 per cent carbohydrates. Therefore it does not automatically provide other nutrients the way starchy grains do. Secondly, it adds energy to food without apparently changing its weight or volume but making it more palatable, and therefore promotes obesity. Finally, sticky sweets lead to dental cavities.

9. *Why does a mixture of cereal and pulse protein become a good quality protein?*

   Cereal protein is deficient in the amino acid lysine and pulse protein is deficient in another amino acid called methionine. Since the deficient amino acid in the two proteins is different, they make up for each other's deficiency.

10. *What are the special benefits of soya bean?*

    Soya bean has a unique composition – high protein and high fat – but no special benefits. It is an acceptable food, but its higher protein content is not essential for meeting our protein needs.

11. *Which cooking oil is the best?*

    Scientific knowledge on this subject has travelled full circle. The best oils according to current knowledge are some of the traditional oils – mustard oil and soyabean oil. Along with these a small amount of saturated fat such as coconut oil, butter, ghee or palmolein would give the currently recommended ratio of 1:1:1 for saturated, monounsaturated and polyunsaturated fatty acids (PUFA), and also provide a reasonable ratio of n-6 : n-3 PUFA.

It is often asked how beneficial olive oil is. Olive oil is rich in monounsaturated fatty acids. Its effect on blood cholesterol level is essentially neutral – it neither raises nor lowers the level. As one of the oils in the diet, it is acceptable. But neither is it essential, nor it is desirable as the sole oil in the diet. And certainly, one should not take olive oil in the hope of any miraculous health benefits.

12. *What is cholesterol?*

Cholesterol is a normal constituent of the body and performs important functions. It can be obtained from the diet and can also be synthesised in the body. There is a mechanism in the body which ensures that if we do not take enough cholesterol in the diet, the body manufactures it to make up the deficit; on the other hand if we take too much cholesterol in the diet, cholesterol synthesis in the body is suppressed. But this mechanism has limits, and it is not equally efficient in all of us. The excess of dietary cholesterol leads to accumulation of cholesterol in the body, which shows up in a higher level of blood cholesterol. Further, some individuals are specially prone to develop high blood cholesterol.

It is good to remember that eggs are the single largest source of cholesterol in the Indian diet. One egg contains about 250 mg of cholesterol, all of which is in the yellow of the egg. *No food of plant origin contains any cholesterol.* Therefore, in an otherwise vegetarian diet, one egg per day still leaves the cholesterol intake within the permissible level of 300 mg. Whether one can tolerate this level of intake without a rise in blood cholesterol can best be found out by measuring the blood cholesterol level before and after four weeks of an-egg-a-day routine. If there is no significant difference between the two levels, the person can take an egg everyday if he likes.

However, if the level rises after four weeks of taking eggs, the person should stop taking eggs (he may still take the white of the egg if he is very keen).

The amount of cholesterol in the diet is not the only determinant of blood cholesterol. Saturated dietary fats (eg butter and ghee) also raise the blood cholesterol whereas unsaturated dietary fats (most of the vegetable oils) lower the blood cholesterol. However, that does not mean the more unsaturated the fat the better. Lop-sided diets having only unsaturated fats such as corn oil or sunflower oil may lower cholesterol, but they also lower immunity, and increase the tendency of the blood to clot. Therefore, as discussed above, saturated and unsaturated fat both have a place in the diet.

13. *What is the place of nuts in a balanced diet?*

First, nuts are not essential in a balanced diet. Secondly, nuts provide about 6 calories per gram because of their high fat content. Thirdly, walnut and almonds are more heart-friendly than other nuts, provided we do not eat too many. To prevent weight gain, it might help to know that 12 walnut-halves, 12 almonds or 20 peanuts weigh 25 grams, and give about 150 calories – compare it with the energy content of other foods in Table 2 to decide how much to cut down on the chapattis or some other foods to prevent weight gain. Alternatively, a brisk 25-minute walk will burn off 150 calories: in short, a one-minute walk will compensate for one gram of nuts.

14. *Is fruit juice better than the fruit?*

No, the rat's tail cannot be longer than the rat even if it seems so. Fruit contains the juice, and in addition the fibre.

15. *Are multivitamin tablets necessary?*

No, strictly speaking it is possible to get enough vitamins from a balanced diet. Further, taking the tablets may induce a false sense of security. This is an important consideration because natural foods such as fruits and vegetables provide not only vitamins and minerals but also nutrients which are not yet scientifically well established but may be important as anti-infective, anti-cancer and antioxidant agents.

However, in spite of these considerations, if one is in a state of enhanced vitamin requirement (eg stress, illness, antibiotic treatment), along with a balanced diet, one can take a multivitamin tablet containing only physiological doses (not mega doses) of vitamins. It may do some good, and certainly does no harm.

16. *'An apple a day keeps the doctor away'. What does this mean?*

The guarantee is supported neither by science nor experience. In any case, it may not even be desirable to keep entirely away from doctors. Doctors not only treat those who are ill, they also help healthy people grow healthier.

17. *What is the nutritional value of soft drinks?*

A bottle of aerated soft drink provides 50-80 calories in the form of sugar. It also contains caffeine or related chemicals, which may help keep us awake in spite of fatigue (also see Chapter 4). Carbon dioxide gas, which is responsible for the fizz, has no appreciable physiological significance.

18. *Is alcohol good for the heart?*

This is still not well established but alcohol is certainly bad for the liver. It seems wine may do some good to the heart because of its antioxidant content, but not because of its alcohol content. It is preferable to get antioxidants from fruits and vegetables rather than from alcohol (also see Chapter 4).

4

All Style, No Substance

One reason why I don't drink is because I wish to know when I am having a good time.

NANCY ASTOR

It is unfortunate that in today's consumerist society, living in style is synonymous with a lifestyle that lacks substance, but includes substances that have no role in providing sustenance. The icons of our society are film stars and sportspersons, and many of them endorse products that are, at best, irrelevant to a healthy lifestyle. In this chapter we shall consider some substances which contribute virtually nothing of value to our diet but are yet consumed in a substantial quantity by a substantial number of people. Further, they are consumed by people who know that these substances may be harmful. They still consume them to conform, to socialise, and to get temporary but quick and easy relief from fatigue, anxiety, boredom or stress. Therefore, the surest way to give up these substances is to live a life in which these reasons will either cease to exist or cease to matter.

CAFFEINE

Caffeine is a pharmacologically active ingredient of tea, coffee, cola drinks and chocolate. It stimulates the nervous system. As a result, it generally relieves fatigue and boredom. It also improves physical and mental performance if it has been impaired due to exhaustion or lack of sleep. But it cannot improve mental performance if it has not been already impaired. However, it may improve physical performance even if the baseline is optimum for the individual. But for such a genuine improvement in physical performance, the dose of caffeine required exceeds the permissible limit for athletes, and might therefore lead to disqualification.

The downside of the stimulant effect is that caffeine might make a person anxious, agitated, jittery or irritable. Therefore, caffeine-containing drinks do not improve performance if it has deteriorated as a result of anxiety. Rather, in such cases the performance might deteriorate further; people with unsteady hands become more unsteady under the influence of these drinks. The alertness produced by the drinks might become undesirable if taken close to bedtime. The degree to which they postpone sleep varies enormously from person to person. Caffeine always increases the heart rate, and might induce palpitation or irregularity of the heart beat. It might constrict coronary arteries, which can be dangerous if the arteries are already partially blocked by fatty deposits. It also stimulates acid secretion in the stomach, which may aggravate a peptic ulcer.

In healthy persons, long-term effects of caffeine depend a lot on the quantity consumed regularly. Moderate quantities seem to be essentially harmless. Heavy intake has been linked to heart disease, breast cancer, and spontaneous abortions, but the evidence is weak and controversial. That is why so many can consume caffeine-containing drinks regularly throughout life, and get away with it!

Behavioural effects

Caffeine-containing drinks bring welcome alertness and elevation of mood within a few minutes. On top of that, the drinks taste good and smell good. But within an hour or two, the effect of caffeine wears out, and the person gets more tired than before. The 'solution' is simple: one more cup of the same. The cycle repeats itself. The result is that by the evening the person is tired, irritable and jittery, and even caffeine does not help much. As Dean Ornish says, caffeine does not give energy, it borrows energy from the future. However, the temptation to get a bout of energy is so irresistible that the person ends up taking a few cups everyday. Finally, the person is addicted to tea or coffee. If denied his dose at the usual time, he not only misses it, he gets a real headache which is relieved only by caffeine. Further, the person develops tolerance to caffeine; he gradually needs more and more quantity of caffeine to get the same effect.

Facts and figures

In general, coffee has the maximum amount of caffeine, tea and cola drinks intermediate amounts, and chocolates the least (Table 4.1). It is quite illogical that although tea and cola drinks have nearly the same amount of caffeine, children are usually denied tea but not cola drinks[1]. Decaffeinated tea and coffee have only negligible amounts of caffeine. The caffeine content of herbal 'tea' depends on whether, in addition to other herbs, it also has tea[2]. If one must have caffeine-containing drinks, one should ensure that the caffeine intake is restricted to safe limits (Table 4.2).

---

[1] Happily children are now being discouraged from having even cola drinks.
[2] Tea is also a herb.

Table 4.1. CAFFEINE CONTENT OF DRINKS AND CHOCOLATE

Item	Caffeine content
1 cup coffee	100 mg
1 cup tea	50 mg
1 Coke/Pepsi	40 mg
1 dark chocolate bar, 35 g	15 mg
1 milk chocolate bar, 35 g	5 mg
1 cup chocolate milk	5 mg

Table 4.2. RELATIVE SAFETY OF CAFFEINE

Relative safety	Daily intake (mg)	Items
Safe	100	1 cup of coffee or 2 cups of tea
Moderately safe	200-300	2-3 cups of coffee[3]
Undesirable	>500	5 cups of coffee
Toxic	>1000	10 cups of coffee[4]

Protective effects of tea, coffee and chocolate

During the last decade or so, there has been plenty of research on tea, coffee and chocolate, largely sponsored, directly or indirectly, by the respective industries, which has shown these products to be protective against several diseases, particularly heart disease and cancer. What this research has found is perfectly true, *but* it is only part of the truth. The protective effect has been attributed to the antioxidants in these 'foods', not to the caffeine. Further,

---

[3] Two or three cups of coffee in one go can help improve one's athletic performance. Taking still larger quantities does not improve the performance further.

[4] Ten cups of coffee lets off serious neural symptoms such as a humming sound in the ears, visual hallucinations and numbness in the limbs.

antioxidants are found not only in tea, coffee and chocolates, but in plant foods in general. A person taking adequate amounts of fruits and vegetables, and also spices, does not have to tolerate the ill-effects of caffeine for the sake of antioxidants.

Alternatives to tea, coffee and cola drinks

Tea, coffee and cola drinks may not be essential dietary items, and may even be slightly harmful, but they serve a vital role in social intercourse. Tea and coffee are only an excuse to meet, and add charm and value to the meeting. Sitting down to eat something together is a sign of equality, friendship and intimacy, and tea or coffee fulfil this role in a rather convenient and inexpensive manner. That is why 'let us meet over a cup of tea' is such a common expression. But there is no dearth of healthy alternatives to tea, coffee and cola drinks. In a way, the healthiest alternative is water. But since 'just water' has social limitations, a few other alternatives have been listed in Table 4.3.

Table 4.3. ALTERNATIVES TO TEA, COFFEE AND COLA DRINKS

Hot drinks	Cold drinks
Herbal tea	Lemonade (Nimboo-paani)
Kaiser-ilaichi milk	Fruit juices and squashes
Badam milk	Ginger ale
Sherbat-milk	Jal-jeera
Malt	Lassi/buttermilk

Herbal tea

Although several commercial formulations of herbal tea are readily available, it can also be made easily at home from basic ingredients. Boil cardamom (*ilaichi*), clove (*laung*), ginger (*sundh*), black pepper (*kali mirch*), tulsi leaves and wheat bran (*choker*) in water – all of these are not essential – just two or three ingredients will also do. Very small quantities of the ingredients suffice because of their strong aroma. The drink may be sweetened with sugar, jaggery (*gur*) or honey. Milk may also be added, if desired.

Malt

Malt is a very delicious and nutritious drink, although a little cumbersome to prepare.[5] Germinate *jowar*, *bajra* and *ragi*. Blend the germinated grains with milk, water and jaggery. Boil, and serve hot.

Ginger ale

Extract the juice from 100 g of ginger. Make a syrup by boiling half a kg of sugar in half a litre of water. Add the ginger juice to the syrup and mix. Add half a cup (about 100 ml) of fresh sour lime juice and mix. When cool, add two pinches of sodium benzoate (preservative), and bottle it. A bottle of ginger ale concentrate is ready. Dilute 10-20 ml of the concentrate with cold water to make a drink.[6]

ALCOHOL

Everybody knows alcohol is bad, yet people have been drinking for millennia. Although many drink in order to drown sorrows of the past and worries about the future in the euphoria of the present, that is not the only reason. People also drink to celebrate special occasions, to party, and to be a part of the crowd rather than stand apart. Finally, an addict drinks because he has to

---

[5] Once the procedure is streamlined, it is not very cumbersome. Swami Vivekananda Kendra, Bangalore, prepares malt for a few hundred persons twice a day round the year.

[6] Source: *Yoga and Total Health*, July 2000, p.18

drink: he needs no other reason. The fact is that drinking is a part of the lifestyle of many, and their number is growing rapidly, especially among the youth. Therefore, we need to discuss this issue dispassionately and in some detail.

The biological effects of alcohol

What alcohol does to the human body depends heavily on the quantity and frequency of consumption, but a certain amount of generalisation is possible. The biological effects of alcohol may be divided into acute and long-term effects.

Acute effects

Acute effects are those which are seen soon after a drink.

Alcohol is a central nervous system depressant[7]. The parts of the brain which are most susceptible to the depressant effect are those which are most highly evolved. These parts deal with speech, memory, discrimination, comprehension, judgement and abstract thinking. Since these parts are depressed, not only is the memory or capacity to understand impaired and the speech affected, the restraint which higher parts of the brain impose on basic instincts and impulses is also weakened. As a result, a person may become garrulous, abusive, quarrelsome, violent or indiscreet. Thus the apparent 'stimulation' of the person is due to depression of those parts of the brain which normally suppress undesirable behaviour. However, if the person continues to drink more, the depressant effect spreads to relatively primitive parts of the brain as well. As a result, the person's seeing, hearing and gait are affected. Finally the person becomes unconscious. Once consciousness is lost, it takes very little additional alcohol to depress the respiratory and heart

---

[7] This may appear surprising because alcohol apparently activates a person. The paradox has been explained in the next few lines.

centres. When that happens, breathing and heart beat may stop and the person dies. However, this is not how alcohol usually kills. A more common way is that the person vomits. Since the reflexes which normally prevent the vomitus from entering the windpipe are depressed, part of the vomitus enters the lungs, which in turn makes breathing laboured and ineffective. Finally the person may get suffocated and die. The commonest route by which alcohol kills is, however, by acting as a slow poison. Over years, it leads to liver disease or some other fatal ailment: these are long term effects.

Some other acute effects of alcohol continue into the night, the next day, and sometimes for weeks following an evening of heavy drinking. Sleep during the night after drinking is disturbed. When the person gets up, he has a 'hangover' characterised by headache, anxiety or depression, excessive thirst, and an upset stomach. Finally, following a night of heavy drinking, abstract thinking may remain impaired *for up to one month*: this is particularly important for students to know.

Long-term effects

Alcohol is, first and foremost, a central nervous system depressant. In those who have been drinking for several years, the size and weight of the brain are smaller, especially on the left side – the side which is more involved in language, logic and mathematics. Besides, sleep disturbance is common, and there may be loss of memory, dementia or even frank psychosis[8]. With prolonged use, tolerance is common, which means that the person needs progressively larger amounts of alcohol to produce the same degree of euphoria.

By far the commonest and most predictable serious consequence of prolonged use of alcohol is liver disease: generally cirrhosis, and sometimes cancer of the liver. This is a progressive, essentially

---

[8] Psychosis is a mental illness in which the patient is not in touch with reality.

incurable, and eventually a fatal problem. Digestive organs other than the liver are also commonly affected: indigestion, heart burn, chronic pancreatitis and gastrointestinal cancers are fairly frequent among habitual drinkers. Absorption of calcium from the intestines is impaired, thereby increasing the risk of osteoporosis.

A highly predictable consequence of chronic alcoholism is high blood pressure. High blood pressure, in turn, very significantly increases the risk of getting a stroke. The relationship between alcohol and coronary heart disease is U-shaped (Fig. 4.1), which means that while a small amount of alcohol might somewhat reduce the risk of heart disease, larger amounts definitely increase the risk. Further, alcohol might also induce another incurable form of heart disease which affects the heart muscle itself, called cardiomyopathy. The myopathy extends to other muscles of the body too, giving rise to progressive weakness.

Prolonged use of alcohol affects reproductive function adversely in both men and women. In men, it results in impotence; in women, it affects pregnancy. Alcohol consumption by the mother increases significantly the possibility of facial abnormalities, mental retardation, and attention deficit hyperactivity disorder in the child. Alcohol may also be passed on to the baby through the mother's milk, and thereby affect the baby even after pregnancy. Therefore, alcohol is a strict no-no for women during pregnancy and lactation. Alcohol also increases the risk of a woman getting breast cancer.

Alcohol also has some generalised effects on health. It suppresses immunity directly, and also indirectly by inducing malnutrition. The reason why an alcoholic generally gets malnourished is that alcohol itself provides seven calories per gram, and therefore taking too much alcohol reduces the need for calories from other foods. However, calories from alcohol are 'empty calories': they are not associated with a supply of protein or vitamins. Further, alcoholic drinks are expensive. Therefore, a compulsive drinker often squanders much of his income on alcohol, and cannot afford a nutritious diet. The end result is overall poor health.

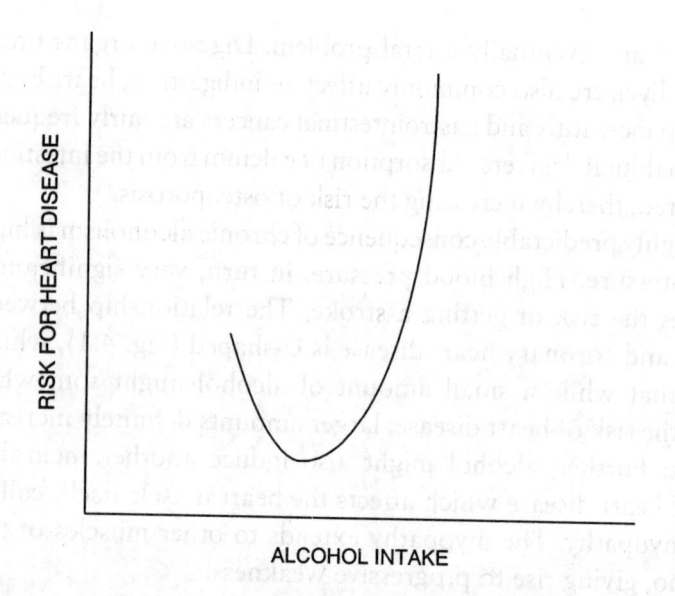

[Graph: Risk for Heart Disease (y-axis) vs Alcohol Intake (x-axis), U-shaped curve]

Fig. 4.1. *The relationship between alcohol intake and risk for coronary heart diseases is U-shaped. While a small regular intake might reduce the risk, a larger intake definitely increases the risk. However, even a small intake is not recommended for reasons discussed in the text.*

The long-term effects of alcohol might get reversed in early cases if further alcohol intake is stopped. But in advanced cases, even if further consumption of alcohol is stopped, it may be possible at best to halt further deterioration; in several cases, the condition may continue to deteriorate.

Behavioural effects of alcohol

The behavioural effects of alcohol are well known and are of great importance to the individual, his family, and the society. These effects arise primarily from the effects of alcohol on the nervous system. As mentioned earlier, alcohol depresses the central nervous system. Depression of the restraint imposed by the 'thinking part' of the brain on crude behaviour leads to a release phenomenon.[9] As a result, the person no longer feels any inhibition about being vulgar and violent. The brunt of this change is usually borne by the wife and children. Alcohol is the leading cause of domestic violence. It also encourages criminal tendencies: people are known to get drunk before committing a crime, because they know that will make it easier. Sometimes the person himself is the victim of this tendency: the rate of suicide among alcoholics is higher than among the general population. An important consequence of the acute effects of alcohol is rash driving, leading to road accidents. Driving needs quick decisions based on continuously changing information, and steady limbs. Both these abilities are seriously impaired by alcohol. To make matters worse, the person's confidence in his abilities may be unrealistically high. The long term effects of alcohol on behaviour eventually ruin relationships with family and friends, and at the workplace. The person may eventually use alcohol as a substitute for relationship. But since it cannot fulfil that role, the person may go into depression and even commit suicide. But, more often, the person is brought to his senses by chronic liver disease or some other serious physical problem. Unfortunately that happens too late for recovery from the disease, and the person spends the last few years of his life knocking in vain at the doors of all sorts of doctors and hospitals.

Everyone knows what the end of overindulgence in alcohol could be, and yet so many just cannot stop themselves. The excuses are generally sought in the circumstances – the family, working environment, the circle of friends, and so on. But the person himself has to assume responsibility and save himself. Others, including doctors, can only help and guide. Sometimes an escape is sought through the genes. While there is a tendency to inherit a liking for alcohol, there is always the choice to use

---

[9] To visualise this, consider the release phenomenon school children display when the teacher is not in the classroom.

that as an excuse and succumb to the craving, or to consider that a strong reason for not touching alcohol. There are people who use their knowledge of this genetic weakness of theirs to keep away from alcohol altogether because they fear that once they sip it, they might be unable to stop.

How much, if at all

There is reasonable agreement on how much alcohol might be generally taken without doing any serious harm. Beer is rather dilute, and men are permitted up to two glasses (about 200 ml each) in a day. Wine is a little more concentrated, and therefore only one glass may be taken. Whisky and other concentrated spirits are generally diluted with water or soda before drinking. Up to two such glasses may be taken, each glass containing about 30 ml of the concentrated spirit. Women have a relative deficiency of the enzyme which metabolises alcohol. Therefore, their tolerance levels are lower. Hence women are permitted only half the amount, that is up to one glass of beer or half a glass of wine or one peg of whisky per day. During pregnancy and lactation it is advisable not to take even this amount because of the effects of alcohol on the baby as discussed earlier.

What has been said above *does not mean* that a certain quantity of alcohol should be taken. Those who do not already take it should stay away from it and those who do should also at least bring the quantity down to the levels mentioned above. Further, alcohol should not be taken at all, in any quantity, by those who have high blood pressure, irregular heart beat (arrhythmias), liver disease, peptic ulcer, sleep apnea, or breast cancer. Those on medication should also check whether alcohol interacts dangerously with the drugs they are taking. Some such interactions with commonly taken drugs have been listed below.

All sleeping pills and anti-anxiety pills (tranquillisers) depress the nervous system, just like alcohol. Since they work in the same direction, their effects can add up. The result could be such severe depression of breathing as to kill the person. Some drugs used for epilepsy, diarrhoea, fungal infections, and as blood thinners (anticoagulants) also have undesirable interactions with alcohol. A certain variety of antidepressants (MAO inhibitors) interacts with alcohol to raise the blood pressure, and the rise could be high to cause brain hemorrhage and death. Antihistamines, taken for common cold, also depress the nervous system, and may interact sufficiently with alcohol to induce drowsiness, or at least make driving dangerous. Aspirin, taken so commonly for headaches, acts in the same direction as alcohol does on the stomach. Therefore, the two taken together may cause massive bleeding in the stomach.

Does alcohol have a protective effect?

Following the observation popularly known as the French paradox (the French drink wine but suffer less from heart disease), there has been a considerable amount of research on the possibility of alcohol having a protective effect. The results of the research have been conflicting. On one hand, alcohol does increase the blood level of HDL (good) cholesterol, and also promotes the dissolution of clots. On the other hand, alcohol increases the fraction HDL_3 of HDL, and not HDL_2 which is the protective fraction. Further, it has been argued that the apparent protective effect of alcohol may be because in some people it is a way of connecting socially and reducing stress. Another indirect contribution to the protective effect might be made by the antioxidants present in wine.

Putting all the facts known so far together, there is no good case for recommending alcohol for its protective effect. Instead of depending on the antioxidants of wine, it is better to get the antioxidants directly from grapes and other fruits and vegetables. Alcohol can hardly add to the protection offered by a prudent diet and exercise, but can certainly increase the risk of liver disease and several other problems discussed earlier.

Managing socially

One may not like to drink, but there may be social situations in which it becomes impossible to avoid alcohol altogether. In these situations, a few strategies are helpful in minimising its intake. One may drink water or some other substitute available. When forced to have some alcohol, one may add more water and less alcohol. Or, one may indicate a special preference for a 50-50 mixture of beer and soda/7-up/Sprite. Finally, once a glass has been accepted, one should ensure that it does not finish, by sipping it slowly and by replenishing it frequently with water.

Giving it up

Alcohol is an addicting substance. Therefore, giving it up is difficult, and withdrawal causes physical symptoms such as nausea, sweating, anxiety and trembling. Withdrawal should, therefore, be preferably under medical supervision.

As important as giving up alcohol is to stay away from it. An important factor which compels one to keep coming back is the control it gives the individual over managing stress. Without having to depend on the understanding and love of others around and without having to visit a counsellor, the person is able to get some relief from stress. But alcohol does not eliminate stress – it provides only temporary relief just as caffeine suspends fatigue temporarily.[10] The spiritual worldview gives the ideal solution: it enables the individual to eliminate stress without depending on anybody or anything, and it has no harmful effects. If one goes through the principles of Alcoholics Anonymous (AA), a

---

[10] However, unlike caffeine, alcohol does not improve any type of performance. Its beneficial effect on social skills is illusory. It cannot build any lasting relationships based on love and trust; however, it can destroy many.

self-help group which helps people give up alcohol and stay away from it, one will see that they are not unlike the principles of spiritual life.

SMOKING

Television bulletins on environmental pollution have made us all familiar with poisonous gases and particulate matter concentrations approaching or crossing acceptable limits in metropolitan cities. Smokers watching television probably do not realise that each time they smoke, they voluntarily expose themselves to smoke which has a particulate matter concentration 500,000 times higher than in the most polluted city in the world. Further, cigarette smoke has a carbon monoxide concentration which is 800 times higher than the upper limit considered acceptable, and a mixture of about 5000 chemicals, many of which are known to increase the risk of causing cancer. Not only the smoker, but even his wife, children and others around him are exposed to high levels of pollutants several times a day through the smoke he blows into the air that they breathe. According to a recent survey, twenty-one per cent of adult Indians smoke.[11] If we add their non-smoking families and colleagues, it amounts to about half the population and hence all efforts at reducing environmental pollution become completely redundant.

Why people smoke

Most smokers may not be aware of how polluted the smoke they inhale is, which they make their near and dear ones also inhale, but they all know that smoking is bad for health. Why do they smoke then, and continue to do so?

---

[11] *The Hindu* – CNN-IBN State of the Nation Survey. *The Hindu*, 14 August 2006, page 12.

Most smokers start quite young, usually in their teens. The initiation is often through a persuasive offer made by a close friend. The curiosity to try something new, the urge to conform, and an attitude of defiance – all so characteristic of youth – combine to make the 'victim' try his first cigarette or *bidi*. The effects of the first cigarette are not very pleasant: dizziness, light-headedness, a violent fit of coughing and even vomiting. But the young boy has a tendency to suppress and ignore these so that he is not labelled a 'sissy' or a kid. He puts up a brave front, and tries the second, and then the third cigarette. Unfortunately, tolerance to smoking develops rapidly, and soon the boy starts enjoying it – he enjoys being part of the crowd, he enjoys the stylish way he holds the cigarette and blows smoke, and he enjoys the pleasant effects of nicotine. Nicotine reduces anxiety and pain, improves concentration and memory, and helps lose weight. Depending on the dose, it can relax a tense individual, or arouse a depressed one; and smokers learn through experience how to vary their style of smoking to get the desired effect. These pleasant effects hook the young boy to smoking, but he soon discovers that 'not smoking' not only deprives him of the pleasant effects but causes headaches, anger, irritability, restlessness and disturbed sleep. Now he is addicted to smoking, and depends on smoking to keep the unpleasant effects away. Thus, what starts as a social activity and youthful adventure ends up as a biological dependence on a potentially lethal practice.

Effects of smoking

Smoking has numerous effects because it exposes the body to at least three agents: the nicotine in tobacco, the smoke, and the heat.

Effects of nicotine

Smoking is an extremely efficient drug delivery system. Nicotine starts entering the blood as soon as one starts to smoke. Its effects on the brain are responsible for the changes in mood and performance which compel the person to smoke cigarettes one after another at progressively shorter intervals. Further, nicotine paralyses the tiny hair (called cilia) which line the air passages. These normally keep sweeping upwards the dust and other particles present in the air that we breathe in, and thereby prevent these particles from entering the lungs. Nicotine also constricts the blood vessels. The effect is widespread, but may produce specially undesirable effects in a few organs of the body. It may cause angina or even a heart attack. In the brain, the reduction in blood supply may lead to a stroke. It affects the legs, and may cause pain while walking. In extreme cases, it may eventually affect the tissues in the legs. The dead tissues (gangrene) generally get infected, necessitating amputation. Reduced blood supply due to smoking may lead to back pain. Blockage of blood flow to the penis might lead to impotence in men.

Effects of the smoke

Smoke is a complicated mixture having thousands of chemicals. One of these, which produces an immediate effect, is carbon monoxide.[12] Carbon monoxide competes very powerfully with oxygen for combining with haemoglobin. As a result, the presence of very small quantities of carbon monoxide is sufficient to reduce the oxygen carrying capacity of blood substantially. On one hand, the blood supply has been reduced by the constriction of blood vessels brought about by nicotine and on the other hand, the amount of oxygen carried by blood is reduced by carbon monoxide. The result is that if the oxygen supply to a vital organ like the heart is already restricted due to coronary artery disease, smoking can trigger a heart attack.

---

[12] Carbon monoxide is the gas which sometimes kills people who sleep in a closed room with burning coal inside.

Besides carbon monoxide and other gases, cigarette smoke has a lot of particulate matter. As mentioned earlier, the concentration of such matter in cigarette smoke is several thousand times greater than that in the air in highly polluted cities. A non-specific acute effect of such a high density of particles is an increase in airway resistance. In other words, it takes more effort to breathe in and breathe out, a situation similar to that in an asthmatic attack.

As the smoke goes in, its particulate matter condenses in the lungs to form a thick sludge called tar. Tar is a rich mixture of cancer producing substances called carcinogens.

Effects of heat

The temperature of cigarette smoke as it forms is about 1000^0C, i.e. ten times the temperature of boiling water. It is amazing that people voluntarily expose their mouth and throat to so much heat. Repeated exposure to so much heat is itself enough to increase the risk of cancer of the mouth and throat, to which may be added the effects of hundreds of carcinogenic chemicals in cigarette smoke.

Health consequences of smoking

There is no smoker who does not know that smoking harms him. Yet most smokers continue to smoke because, on one hand, the pull is too strong to resist; and on the other hand is the wishful thinking that somehow 'I will escape'. The ill-effects of smoking are not a question of luck. One might escape lung cancer, but that is not the only disease linked to smoking. Further, some ill-effects follow smoking as predictably as the night follows the day. Thus, nobody really escapes. And, it is not a question of 'how many cigarettes a day'. There is a health-cost to be paid, for every cigarette smoked (even if the cigarette is free!)

> **THE FIRE THAT FOLLOWS THE SMOKE**
>
> - Smoking is the leading preventable cause of chronic disease.
> - The link between smoking and cardiovascular disease is as well established as that between smoking and lung cancer.
> - To smoking may be attributed:
>   - 80% of the deaths due to lung cancer.
>   - 80% of the cases of emphysema.
>   - 75% of coronary heart disease in young adults who are otherwise at low risk.
>   - 30% of all deaths due to cancer.
>   - 30% of all deaths due to coronary heart disease.
>   - 20% of all cardiovascular diseases.

Cardiovascular disease

Smoking is a major risk factor for cardiovascular diseases such as high blood pressure, angina, myocardial infarction, stroke and peripheral vascular diseases. Smoking increases the chances of getting these diseases significantly and consistently through several mechanisms, the end result of which is the accelerated development of atherosclerosis. Further, smoking can superimpose some acute changes to precipitate myocardial infarction or a stroke. To some extent, the blocking of arteries by atherosclerosis is a universal consequence of aging, and it occurs at an earlier age in smokers. But due to the physiological reserves that we have, atherosclerosis often proceeds silently for several decades. However, during smoking, a few things happen which can upset the delicate balance on which the well-being of the person hinges. First, the carbon monoxide enters the blood, reducing the amount of oxygen delivered, even if the blood flow remains the same. But the blood flow does not remain the same: it falls because nicotine constricts blood vessels. Secondly, smoking makes blood more prone to clot.[13] If a blood vessel is partly blocked, and has narrowed down further due to nicotine, a small clot is enough to block it completely. The end result may be a rather dramatic decrease in oxygen supply to a

---

[13] Incidentally, even a single heavy oily meal does that.

critical organ like the heart or the brain, leading correspondingly to a myocardial infarction or a stroke. That is how a forty-year old, who has always been hale and hearty might get his first heart attack (myocardial infarction) during or just after that party where he eats well and smokes a few cigarettes.

Respiratory disease

It is a fact that although 80 per cent of those who die of lung cancer have been smokers, more than 80 per cent of the smokers do not get lung cancer. But there are other respiratory problems which every smoker gets without fail. Irritation of the airways by particulate matter in the cigarette smoke increases the formation of sticky mucus in the airways. On the other hand, nicotine paralyses the cilia which normally aid in the expulsion of mucus (along with the particles which it has trapped). The result is that the mucus stays in the lungs during the day, making breathing a little difficult. But at night, since the person does not smoke, the cilia recover from paralysis, and start sweeping the mucus up. When the person gets up, he coughs a lot and brings out the mucus: this is the typical white sputum of chronic bronchitis. Every smoker, sooner rather than later, gets chronic bronchitis, coughs and brings out sputum – the symptoms are at their worst on waking up in the morning. The poor cilia of a smoker have to do in less than eight hours of the night much more than what they do in a non-smoker in twenty-four hours. Naturally, there is always pending work to do. The mucus waiting to be cleared from the lungs may get infected, leading to bronchiectasis, with its typically yellow sputum. Further, the hard work which the respiratory system has to do in order for one to breathe through narrow, mucus-clogged airways, leads to air getting trapped in the lungs, giving rise to a barrel-shaped chest.[14] When these lungs

---

[14] Air trapping means that the air breathed out is slightly less than the air breathed in. This occurs because breathing out is more difficult in this situation than breathing in.

are exposed to bouts of explosive coughing every morning, their structure starts breaking down: the medical term for lungs damaged in this fashion is emphysema. Through mechanisms which are beyond the scope of this book, a person with bronciectasis and emphysema develops a set of problems involving not only the lungs but also the heart. The medical name for this combination is chronic obstructive pulmonary disease (COPD). COPD is something every smoker develops if he smokes hard enough and long enough, and COPD is essentially a progressive and incurable condition. If a smoker is lucky enough to escape cancer and coronary heart disease (CHD), COPD is inevitable. Further, if the person has both CHD and COPD, he cannot benefit much from even a bypass surgery because the blocked coronary arteries can be bypassed, but that does not help the emphysematous lungs. That is why, a person having COPD is destined to move slowly but certainly and predictably towards death.[15]

Cancers in organs other than the lungs

Although the cancer best correlated with smoking is lung cancer, the risk for cancer of the foodpipe, pancreas, urinary bladder and kidney, is also significantly increased by smoking.

Women and smoking

Fortunately, smoking among Indian women is less prevalent than among men. However, it is good to know that women who smoke are more likely to be infertile, and to get menopause earlier than women who do not. Further, a woman who smokes during pregnancy is likely to have a miscarriage or a still-birth. Even if the baby is born alive, it is at high risk of sudden death during infancy. Further, the baby may have a birth defect such as cleft lip or a cleft palate which is obvious, or may have poor memory and slow learning ability which are not so obvious.

---

[15] In a sense, that is everybody's destiny – a smoker or non-smoker – but the reader would well understand the difference.

Passive smoking

A person sitting near someone who smokes is also exposed to high concentrations of carcinogenic and other harmful chemicals. Passive smoking particularly affects the family members of

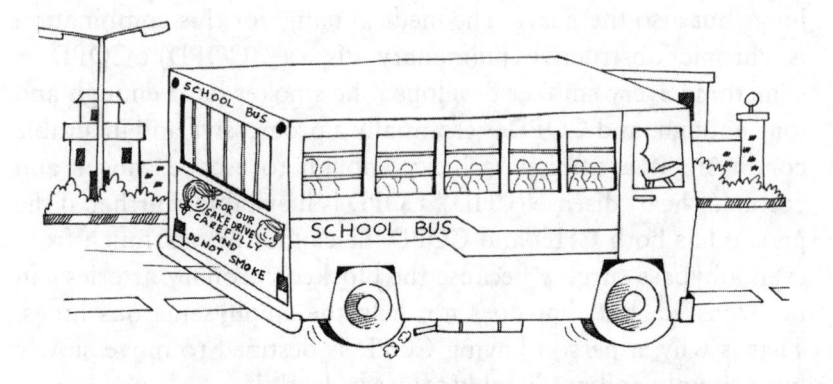

Fig. 4.2. *Even passive smoking increases the risk for lung and heart disease.*

smokers. Passive smoking makes them, particularly children, more prone to cough, colds, bronchial asthma, bronchitis, and even pneumonia. Passive smoking also increases the risk of getting lung cancer and coronary heart disease. (Fig. 4.2).

Going to heaven without actually dying

There are some genuine human needs which smoking satisfies, but the price to be paid is very heavy. Is it possible to satisfy those needs without smoking? The answer is yes: yoga satisfies all those needs. Like smoking, yoga also improves memory and concentration, and helps overcome stress, lethargy, depression and pain. By providing some physical activity and reducing greed for food, yoga also prevents the tendency to be overweight. All these things happen as part of a generalised change in outlook characterised by focus on what is really worthwhile. That process eliminates many of the everyday problems which result from lack of focus, getting engaged in ego hassles and getting attached to sensory pleasures. There is one more important similarity between yoga and smoking which has great psychological significance. In both cases, the person is not dependent on any external agency for his needs. For example, he is not dependent on silence outside for mental concentration, not dependent on his wife or children behaving in a particular manner for remaining stress-free, and not dependent on delicious food for his happiness. Independence from external objects, events, circumstances and people around us for satisfying some basic psychological needs is what makes smoking pleasurable. A person is angry with the child: he lights a cigarette to overcome the anger. A person is hungry: he lights a cigarette to overcome hunger. The flight is delayed: the person lights a cigarette to overcome anxiety. A person feels secure carrying the solution to so many problems in his pocket all the time. During yoga, the person does not even have to have a pocket: he just carries a certain attitude in his head and heart, and all these problems are solved. And, to enjoy the bliss, the person does not have to die of a dreaded ailment such as CHD, COPD or cancer.

Becoming an ex-smoker

Ex-smokers deserve a great deal of respect because to stay away from smoking is much more difficult for persons who once used to smoke. Apart from the lack of adequate motivation, there are two deterrents which prevent a smoker from even trying to achieve this respectable position. The first of these is the belief that the attempt to quit is bound to fail. The second deterrent is the 'knowledge' that the damage already done by smoking is irreversible. Let us examine both.

It is a fact that most smokers have tried to quit at least once, and about three-fourths are back to smoking within three months. In one study, it was found that less than twenty per cent of the smokers who tried to quit succeeded at the first attempt, another five per cent at the second attempt, another five per cent at the third attempt, another ten per cent after several more attempts. In other words, in spite of so many attempts, less than forty per cent succeeded in quitting. However, an optimistic way of looking at the same data is that a failed attempt is not reason enough to get disheartened: it does not indicate a specific weakness of an individual smoker – it happens to almost every smoker. Secondly, repeated attempts do improve the chances of success. Why should a person assume that he will be among the sixty per cent who might fail even after several attempts – he could equally well be among the forty per cent who do succeed. It has been seen that success rates are high after an event like a heart attack. Why not build up the same will power earlier and escape the attack?

Now let us examine the second deterrent to quitting. Many long-time smokers assume that they have already damaged their lungs and heart beyond repair and giving up now would not help much. According to calculations made by the American Cancer Society, a long-time smoker who quits smoking today lowers his risk for lung cancer to the level of a non-smoker after ten years, and his risk for coronary heart disease comes down to that of a non-smoker in fifteen years. One may find the wait for 10-15 years too long. However, some benefits begin much sooner. The American Cancer Society has also found that within twenty minutes of quitting, the blood pressure may drop to normal; within eight hours carbon monoxide level in the blood returns to normal; within twenty-four hours the possibility of a heart attack goes down; and within forty-eight hours the food tastes and smells much better. The additional risk for lung cancer and heart disease might take 10-15 years to disappear, but the decline begins much earlier: within one year of quitting, the risk for heart diseases is half that of a smoker.

Although there is a grain of truth in both the reasons which smokers often have for not trying to quit, the above discussion shows that the picture is not as bleak as it is sometimes made out to be. Determined efforts to quit do succeed – if not the first time, at a subsequent attempt. Secondly, every smoker benefits from quitting – even a long-time smoker – and several tangible benefits are experienced within two days of quitting.

The process of quitting

There are two ways to quit – one is to reduce the number of cigarettes smoked per day gradually; the other is to simply stop smoking one fine day. Both have their pros and cons, and one can choose the method which suits the personality of the smoker better.

If one chooses the gradual method, it should be kept in mind that the most difficult to give up is the first cigarette of the day. It is better to start with the easier ones. One may use various strategies to achieve a reduction in number: keep a daily record of the number smoked, avoid situations in which there is a tendency to light a cigarette, remove ashtrays from the home and the office, buy only one or two cigarettes at a time instead of a whole packet, smoke only in an unpleasant environment like the bathroom, etc. When a substantial reduction in smoking has been achieved, it is time to give up altogether, including the first cigarette of the day.

If one decides to stop completely all of a sudden, the symptoms of nicotine withdrawal such as irritability, restlessness and headaches are quite likely. These may be reduced by using nicotine patches or nicotine gum in progressively smaller amounts. Relaxation techniques such as meditation or *shavasana* also help in managing the withdrawal symptoms.

Half-hearted attempts to quit smoking are destined for failure. Therefore, one should begin only when mentally prepared for it. Once the decision has been taken, it should be announced to family and friends. That helps in two ways: first, their cooperation helps the process of quitting; secondly, one does not go back on the decision because it involves losing face. If one is not fully confident, professional help of a physician, a psychiatrist or a counsellor may be sought. Finally, failing once does not mean that one will never succeed. One has to find the right combination of strong will-power while the attempt to quit is on, and the optimism to try again if the attempt fails. The first 'guilty cigarette' which spoils an attempt to quit should be treated as an aberration rather than an excuse to say, 'Now my neat record of so many weeks has been spoilt anyway. What is the use continuing to deprive myself.' As Dean Ornish says, quitting smoking is a process, not an event.

The positive way of quitting smoking is to first understand that quitting does not mean giving up a pleasure for the sake of better health or a longer life. Quitting smoking is the first step in replacing an inferior pleasure by a superior pleasure. To get the logic of this assertion, one has to examine the root of the problem. People generally smoke either to reduce stress or to improve mental performance. If both these ends, and a lot more, are achieved through yoga, the reasons for smoking disappear. If the reasons for smoking disappear, 'not smoking' is not a deprivation any more. Therefore, a comprehensive change in lifestyle, as in yoga, is easier than just giving up smoking. If one decides to just give up smoking, leaving the rest of life and the attitude to life unchanged, it would be natural to view the process as a deprivation. But a yogic change in attitude makes it a pleasant experience to live without smoking, just as it makes it possible to enjoy vegetarian food, take some exercise, and develop a relationship of love and intimacy with the people around us. Thus a one-step reset button is all we need to press in order to experience a total transformation. The transformation would include getting weaned from smoking as a part of the package.

In short, no matter how long a person has been smoking, there is hope. There is no need to regret the past, which is dead and gone, and which nobody can change. The future is still ours, and we can make it better than our past by doing something *now*.

5

Staying Mobile

The sovereign invigorator of the body is exercise, and of all exercises, walking is the best.
                                            THOMAS JEFERSON

While introducing the subject of exercise, Dean Ornish makes the interesting point that exercise is a form of punishment in schools. No wonder, once out of school, we do not like to exercise in spite of knowing that it is good for health. There are certain types of exercise we cannot avoid if they are a part of our occupation or household duties. But for many of us such compulsory exercise does not amount to much. In that case, we exercise only if we voluntarily spend some of our leisure time on either a game like badminton (recreational exercise), or some other physical activity undertaken for the sake of exercise itself. The division between recreational exercise and 'serious' exercise is arbitrary: far from being a punishment, all kinds of physical exercise are potentially enjoyable.

BENEFITS OF EXERCISE

Exercise is potentially enjoyable, but only potentially so. The fact is that most people do not want to exercise unless they have to. Therefore, it helps build up motivation to exercise if one is conscious of the good it does. From a physiological point of view, when we are sitting and doing some mental work or watching TV, our body needs only a limited amount of energy, our heart and lungs do not have to work hard to deliver the limited amount of oxygen to different parts of the body required for generating the required energy, and our muscles are inactive. When we exercise, some of our muscles become active, these muscles need more energy, and to supply this energy, the heart and lungs have to work harder. But those of us engaged in sedentary occupations seldom utilise this capacity of the heart, lungs and muscles to put in extra work. The result is that organs become lazy, and over time lose their capacity for additional work. On the other hand, in physically active individuals, the capacity for additional work is not only retained, but can even improve. A person whose job is sedentary may hold this additional capacity in reserve most of the time, but that does not matter. Possessing reserve capacity helps in coping up with emergencies, and also comes in handy if one is ill. After the age of about thirty, a gradual decline in the reserve is normal. But the rate of this decline can be slowed down remarkably by regular physical activity. This seems to be a global effect: one might say that regular physical activity slows down the process of aging. The long list of benefits of exercise basically derives from the improvement in cardio-respiratory fitness it confers and from the slowing down of the age-related decline in physiological functions.

Moving all mobile parts of the body on a regular basis makes the body flexible, the muscles stronger, and prolongs the duration for which one may perform a physical activity at a stretch (endurance). The human body is such an amazing machine that the value of these benefits of exercise may not be realised by a sedentary young person for a few decades. But as age catches up, there is a tendency to lose one's balance and fall. A person who has been physically active has strong muscles and a flexible body, and therefore may not have these problems, or develop them much later in life. Further, if such a person does fall, a fracture is less likely because of higher bone mineral density (BMD). A decline in BMD (osteoporosis) is also a part of the aging process, and can be slowed down by regular physical activity. At this point, a few clear statements about BMD are necessary. First, for a good BMD, dietary calcium and physical activity are both equally important. Secondly, the time to build up a good BMD is childhood and youth; after that, one cannot improve upon it. Thirdly, the physical activity which improves BMD is that which involves bones, and the BMD improves selectively in bones around the joints which work against resistance. Therefore, to prevent osteoporosis, the key is to build up a good BMD early in life by taking enough calcium and performing exercises which load several parts of the body. After building up a good BMD in youth comes the role of regular lifelong physical activity and adequate calcium intake in reducing the rate of decline in BMD.

A favourable effect of regular physical activity with extensive ramifications is its effect on body weight and body composition. Although it is true that dietary regulation is a more powerful determinant of body weight than exercise, exercise does count. First, moderate physical activity can restore the energy balance if the imbalance is only marginal. Secondly, physical activity increases energy expenditure not only during exercise, but also during the rest of the day, and also slows down the age-related decline in resting energy consumption. Thirdly, exercise improves body composition, reducing the percentage of fat, and enhancing the percentage contribution of muscle mass to body weight. Finally, exercise has so many benefits that it is imprudent to ignore exercise just because it is possible to maintain normal body weight by dietary regulation. An optimum body weight (which may be achieved without exercise) *and* an optimum body composition (which *cannot* be achieved without exercise) are associated with reduced risk for a wide variety of diseases, notably diabetes and cardiovascular diseases. In terms of biochemical tests, this lower risk is reflected in lower fasting blood glucose, better glucose tolerance, lower total and LDL (bad) cholesterol level, and higher HDL (good) cholesterol level.

It is innate wisdom to seek physical workout to beat a mental breakdown. When we are under acute mental stress, we start pacing up and down, or leave home for a brisk walk.[1] Now the relationship between physical activity and mental health has been placed on a scientific footing by the discovery that exercise releases beta-endorphin in the brain, which in turn, elevates the mood.[2] Surveys have also revealed that those who exercise regularly are not prone to depression.[3] Whether it is because of the relief it provides from mental stress, or because it tires a person out, or possibly both, exercise is also good treatment for sleeplessness (insomnia).

Although the effects of exercise on immunocompetence are slightly complex and somewhat controversial, the general consensus is that moderate physical activity taken regularly improves immunity. That is possibly one of the reasons why physically active persons rarely get a cough, a cold or fever.

All the benefits of exercise are reflected in the observation which has been confirmed by several studies that those who get moderate exercise regularly generally live longer than sedentary individuals (technically, they have a lower all-cause mortality). This in itself may not be very important, but what makes it more

---

[1] A modern variant of this response is to pick up the car and drive rashly, thereby passing on stress to other users of the road.

[2] Endorphins are chemicals similar to morphine. Like morphine, they also relieve pain. As is well known, morphine leads to addiction. The release of endorphins by exercise is possibly the reason why regular exercise may also lead to addiction. Many persons who have a regular exercise regime feel uneasy throughout the day on which they miss their exercise.

[3] It has, however, been argued that those who are depressed are unlikely to take the initiative for exercising. Thus depression may be the cause rather than the effect of physical inactivity.

meaningful is the fact that the years added to life are years full of health and joy.

THE AIMS OF EXERCISE

What a person expects from exercise determines, to some extent, the type and amount of exercise he takes, and how serious a business he makes out of something which should essentially be relaxation. The aims of exercise may be broadly categorised into three: staying healthy, improving physical fitness, and developing specific skills.

Health

Staying healthy or recovering health should be everybody's goal, although exercise serves other aims as well. Fortunately, this is also the simplest goal to realise. It has been found that a regular thirty-minute brisk walk everyday leads to remarkable health benefits. People who practice this or its equivalent have significantly lower all-cause mortality than sedentary persons. Further, making the exercise more strenuous by increasing its duration or severity confers very little additional longevity. It does not mean walking longer is bad. What it means is that you may walk longer if you enjoy it. You do not have to do it to live longer. Therefore, if the aim of exercise is just health, which is true for most of us, we do not need much exercise. A thirty-minute walk does not need any special skills or equipment. It needs an investment of time which we should be able to make even if we think we cannot.

Physical fitness

Physical fitness goes a little beyond health, and refers to the degree of cardio respiratory reserve. Although increasing the severity of exercise beyond that of a thirty-minute brisk walk does not confer additional health benefits, it does offer additional physical fitness.

By challenging the body progressively with exercise which is a little harder than what we are accustomed to, we can stretch the limits of our physical fitness further. Physical fitness is reflected in the resting heart rate. The resting heart rate of athletes is usually on the lower side. Another indicator of physical fitness is the time it takes for the heart rate to return to normal after a given amount of exercise: the more fit a person, the less time it takes for the recovery.

It is natural to think that there is no harm in aiming at better physical fitness alongwith good health. Up to a point, that is quite true. In fact, even a thirty-minute brisk walk everyday will also improve physical fitness in addition to providing health benefits. But beyond a point, there can arise a conflict between fitness and health. We have all heard of several top athletes getting a heart attack at a relatively young age while running. These athletes are physically very fit, but obviously they are not very healthy. The reasons why this happens are complex, but one simple explanation which applies to many such cases runs somewhat like this. The improvement in fitness is achieved through increase in the thickness of the musculature of the heart (hypertrophy). The hypertrophied heart can pump more blood with each beat. This efficient heart which beats slowly but pumps more blood with each beat, however, comes at a cost. The cost is the greater blood flow which its thick walls need. The result is that if a person with such a heart has partly blocked coronary arteries, the imbalance between the blood supply and demand can be precipitated rather easily during exercise when the demand is high. That is why a person might get a heart attack during the athletic event.

Skills

A person who is preparing for competitive sports expects from an exercise programme specific skills such as the ability to run a sprint or a marathon, lift heavy weights, or play a particular game better. Developing these skills needs a specially designed training programme. Any improvement in health or physical fitness resulting from the training is incidental, not the primary goal of the programme. In general, improving the cardiorespiratory reserve, which is important for running a marathon, needs training in aerobic exercises.[4] Improving muscle strength needs use of specific groups of muscles against resistance. Improving the flexibility of the body needs stretching type of exercises. Thus the exercise programme is tailored to the needs of the type of sports in which a person wishes to specialise. Specialised training should begin with a good assessment of the baseline characteristics of the person because, partly due to genetic factors, everybody is not equally capable of excelling in every type of sport. Best results can be achieved if the sport selected is in keeping with the inherent talents of the person. Most of us, of course, would not reach the top in any sport, and that is quite okay. For the ordinary person, improvement in health and a moderate gain in physical fitness are quite adequate as the goals of exercise.

THE NITTY-GRITTIES: EXERCISE PRESCRIPTION

The exercise prescription spells out practical details such as which exercise to take, for how long and how often.

Which exercise?

The most important thing to remember is that any exercise is better than no exercise at all. However, since we have a choice, it is better to make an informed choice. For health and fitness, aerobic exercises are better than anaerobic ones. Aerobic

---

[4] The intensity and duration of aerobic exercises are such that all the oxygen required for performing them can be breathed in essentially during the exercise itself. That is not possible with more intense exercise performed for a short time. In the case of these exercises, called anaerobic, the body incurs an 'oxygen debt', which is 'paid back' by breathing in extra oxygen after the exercise.

exercises are those for which the additional oxygen required can be procured by the body during the exercise itself. Walking, long-distance running, badminton, tennis and yogic postures are examples of aerobic exercises. On the other hand, anaerobic exercises are high-intensity brief exercises, eg, a hundred-metre sprint. These exercises need a lot of additional oxygen, and moreover their duration is too short for the body to adapt to the additional demand. The result is that during the exercise the body incurs an oxygen debt which is paid off after the exercise. Among aerobic exercises, a combination of walking or running and yogic postures is probably the simplest and best choice which improves health, physical fitness, endurance as well as flexibility of the body. However, persons above the age of forty should run only after getting clearance from a doctor. Further, if time is enough only for either walking or yogic postures, the latter is a better choice provided a good yoga teacher is available for the first few days. Yogic postures are better than walking because:

1. A judiciously selected set of 15-20 postures can improve the flexibility of the whole body which walking cannot.
2. A person with a temporary disability of a joint can also do at least a few yogic postures, with the result that regularity is better maintained. On the other hand, injuries which produce these disabilities are also least likely with yogic postures. A person who runs may sometimes sprain an ankle; a person who plays tennis may sprain the shoulder. After such injuries, the exercise has to stop for one or two weeks. If a permanent disability makes even walking difficult, a set of yogic postures which needs only the functional parts of the body can be devised.
3. Although yogic postures are low-intensity exercises, the changes in thoracic and abdominal pressure and fluctuations in oxygen supply (due to breath holding) are comparable to those produced by rather high-intensity non-yogic exercises.

Therefore yogic postures yield health and fitness benefits which are out of proportion to the intensity of effort involved.
4. The sequence of postures is so designed that at the end of the session a person is relaxed rather than tired.
5. The gentle and graceful movements, and the breathing and relaxation techniques incorporated in the session have a soothing effect on the mind.
6. Yogic postures can be performed at home in any loose and comfortable dress (including the night pyjamas). They need no company, and only the bare minimum of preliminaries. For these reasons, heat, cold and rain also need not disturb the regularity of the routine. Thus, although any exercise is better than no exercise at all, all exercises are not alike.

How long?

Thirty minutes of walking is quite satisfactory. Running for ten minutes may be quite enough, but to that should be added about ten minutes of warming up and about ten minutes of cooling down. A session of yogic postures generally takes about an hour, but that includes warming up and cooling down. If one is short of time, the time can be cut short, but warming up, cooling down, and in case of yogic postures, relaxing postures, should not be neglected. The minimum duration of an exercise session – yogic or otherwise – should be about twenty-five minutes, comprising of five minutes of warming up, fifteen minutes of harder exercise, and about five minutes of cooling down. Older people generally need a little longer warm-up time.

A beginner starting exercise after years of sedentary life should also start with a shorter duration (about ten minutes), and increase the duration gradually. Persons having health-related problems such as high blood pressure or heart disease should also begin slowly, and follow their doctor's advice.

How intense should the exercise be?

The intensity of exercise is graded in terms of its energy cost, which in turn is determined from the rate of oxygen consumption, ie the volume of oxygen consumed by the person per minute. A rough but fairly reliable assessment of the intensity of exercise can be obtained from the heart rate during the exercise. The simplest formula to find how hard is hard enough but not too hard is based on the percentage of maximum heart rate (MHR) reached towards the end of the exercise. The MHR for a person is 220 minus age. The target heart rate (THR) during exercise is forty-five to eighty per cent of MHR, depending principally on the health status of the person, and whether the person is at the beginning of an exercise programme or has been in it for some time. For example, the MHR of a fifty year old is 220 − 50 = 170 beats per minute. If he is prescribed exercise at sixty per cent of the MHR, his THR will be 170 x 0.6 = 102 beats per minute. At no point during his walk (or any other exercise he is taking) his heart rate should exceed 102 per minute. The heart rate (HR) is generally taken for 10-15 seconds *immediately* at the end of the exercise. It is difficult to take the HR while exercising. On the other hand, after stopping the exercise, the HR comes down *rapidly*. Therefore, it is important to count the pulse immediately upon stopping the exercise, and count it for only 10-15 seconds. The ten-second count may be multiplied by six, or the 15-second count multiplied by four, to get the HR per minute.

However, sometimes we run into difficulty with this approach. Suppose a sixty-year old person is advised to exercise such that his THR is fifty per cent of the MHR. His MHR = 220 − 60 = 160 per minute. Therefore his THR is 160 x 0.50 = 80 per minute. If his resting HR is also 80 per minute, he cannot exercise at all! Another approach (called the Karvonen equation), although a little complex, does not have this problem, and is even otherwise more reliable. In this approach, a percentage of the heart rate reserve (HRR) is added to the resting HR. Suppose the sixty-year old is advised to exercise such that he encroaches upon fifty per cent of the HRR.

MHR	=	220 − 60	=	160 per minute
Resting HR	=	80 per minute		
HRR	=	160 − 80	=	80 per minute
THR	=	(160 − 80) x 0.5 + 80		
	=	40 + 80		
	=	120 per minute		

Let us take another example. Suppose a forty-year old has been told to encroach upon sixty per cent of the HRR, and suppose his resting heart rate is 70 per minute.

MHR	=	220 − 40	=	180 per minute
HRR	=	180 − 70	=	110 per minute
THR	=	(110 x 0.6) + 70		
	=	66 + 70		
	=	136 per minute		

Hence this person's exercise should be of such an intensity that towards the end of exercise, his heart rate is about 136 per minute or less.

'Towards the end of exercise,' means the end of the phase of vigorous exercise. During cooling down, the heart rate starts coming down: we are interested in the highest steady heart rate during exercise, which may be measured by counting the pulse as soon as possible at the end of the phase of vigorous exercise.

How do we count the pulse?

The pulse may be counted at the front of the wrist towards the thumb-side. If you are right-handed, and have a watch on your left wrist, the simplest thing to do is to place two fingers (index and middle finger) of the left hand over the 'pulse area' of the right hand. There is an instinctive tendency to press the 'pulse area' with the tips of the two fingers. But the pulse is actually felt better if you place the pulp of the two fingers rather gently over the 'pulse area'. If you do as described here, you will be able to have a good look at the watch. Start counting the pulse when the fast-moving 'seconds hand' of the watch reaches a specific point. Keep that point in mind, and count the pulse for ten to fifteen seconds.

Walk and talk

If you find calculating the THR and counting the pulse too cumbersome, there is a simpler alternative. As you might have figured out, the idea behind the tedious task is that the severity of exercise should be such that it is challenging enough to coax the body to improve, and yet not so hard as to be unsafe. Both these ends, particularly the latter, can be met by the 'walk and talk' method, but for that you need a companion. The principle of the method is that you can carry out a conversation comfortably while walking only if you are within your safe limits. When the safe limit is crossed, you get breathless while talking.[5]

How often should we exercise?

The next point in an exercise prescription is the frequency, or how often one is to exercise. Ideally, it should be understood that one must exercise daily. But most of us are likely to be irregular and unless the point is emphasised, slipping is likely to become more frequent than the exercise. Therefore, the prescription emphasises that the exercise should be taken at least five days a week. Although some studies have shown that exercise programmes with a frequency of three days a week are also effective, two points are important in this context. For a three-days-a-week programme to be effective, either the intensity or the duration of exercise, or both, have to be increased. Secondly, many of us might find it easier to maintain regularity if something has to be done everyday rather than on alternate days.

---

[5] A companion may not be necessary for the walk and talk test if you talk on the cell phone as you walk! But this not advisable because talking on the cell phone while walking is risky.

How much exercise is necessary?

The total amount of exercise taken by a person is the product of the duration, intensity and frequency of the exercise. This product, which combines all these three factors, is the most exact determinant of the efficacy of an exercise programme. That is why many different combinations of duration, intensity and frequency may be equally effective in improving cardiorespiratory fitness and adding years to one's life. Thus a thirty-minute daily walk may be taken in three instalments of ten minutes each. Further, a thirty-minute walk everyday or a sixty-minute walk on alternate days may be equally effective.

Having said that, however, a few things should be pointed out. First, there is a limit to this formula. A 200-minute walk every Sunday instead of a thirty-minute walk everyday may give more cramps than health benefits. Secondly, one cannot play around too much with the intensity and duration. Mild exercise does not enhance cardiorespiratory fitness even if the duration is prolonged. Heavy exercise, on the other hand, even for a shorter duration, may be unsafe if the existing health status is not good. Therefore, medical advice and at least the 'walk and talk' test should guide the intensity. The main idea behind pointing out that some flexibility is possible in the duration, intensity and frequency of exercise so long as their product is reasonably constant is that one should not make a rigid ritual out of the exercise schedule. The rigidity robs the exercise programme of its joy. And, the secret of any successful exercise programme is that the person should enjoy it.

Climbing step by step

A sedentary person just starting on an exercise programme should start with only 10-20 minutes of moderate exercise (encroaching on about 40% of HRR) a day, 3-5 days a week. The duration of exercise may be increased by about twenty per cent after every fortnight. At this rate, it is possible to achieve a duration of 30-45 minutes in 3-4 months. The frequency should also by then reach close to seven days a week. After that the intensity of the exercise may be increased, increasing the encroachment on HRR by about five per cent every fortnight, finally stopping any further increase in intensity when either it becomes difficult to talk while exercising, or when eighty-five per cent of the HRR has been encroached upon, whichever is earlier.

These are only general guidelines. Older persons might find it necessary to progress at a slower pace, as might those who have been sedentary for a few decades. Those having any serious illness which compromises the ability for exercise should consult their physician before starting an exercise programme, before increasing the duration or intensity, or if they notice any untoward symptoms such as breathlessness, palpitation, dizziness, sweating, or excessive fatigue during the exercise.

PHYSICAL ACTIVITY FOR THE PHYSICALLY UNWELL

When doctors examine a person, they make use of an abbreviation, NAD, which stands for 'No Abnormality Detected', in their reports. This is a technically correct and safe label because the doctor does not know whether the person is normal; he is sure that he has detected no abnormality. If there is no limit to the time available for examining a person and to the number of tests that can be done on the person, not one but several abnormalities will almost certainly be detected. However, the resilience of the body is so remarkable that none of these abnormalities usually prevents us from going about our daily work comfortably. In short, we may not be perfectly okay, even if we feel so. We can go ahead with not only our daily tasks, but also our daily exercise. Having said that, there are some situations where a little care is in order, and generally we know by instinct when it is so. Therefore, the first important requirement is to understand the language of the body. To some extent, if one exercises with awareness, as in yoga, the exercise itself helps us understand this language. The second important thing is to pay heed to what the body says. These simple acts will prevent us from exercising in acute illnesses such as fever, common cold or diarrhoea. In these situations, 'the body knows best', and it will be foolhardy to persist with the resolve to keep up the exercise schedule. In chronic diseases, besides the guidance available from the body itself, adhering to medical advice is helpful. Some helpful tips in this regard are given below. More information is available in relevant chapters of this book. Finally, let your personal doctor have the last word.

Lung diseases

In chronic diseases of the lung such as chronic bronchitis or bronchial asthma, exercise may be avoided early in the morning, specially in winters, because that is the time when symptoms are most troublesome, and it may worsen. Secondly, it is better to split the total amount of exercise to be taken into a few instalments and spread them out over the day. Finally, following a seven days a week exercise schedule is more important in lung disease than in many other situations.

Hypertension

Exercise should be avoided till the blood pressure has been brought down to less than 200/110 mm Hg. Some of the drugs used for hypertension reduce the heart rate, and inhibit its increase. In such a situation, the heart rate at rest and during exercise should be based on the situation prevailing under medication. The intensity of the exercise should be such as to achieve a target heart rate which encroaches on forty per cent of the HRR to start with, and stepped up gradually to eighty-five percent if the clinical condition permits. Exercises in which the intrathoracic pressure goes up very high, and *kapalabhati* (forceful voluntary hyperventilation) should be avoided.

Coronary heart diseases

A lot depends on how severe the disease is, whether the patient is on medication, has undergone angioplasty or a bypass surgery, or has a pacemaker implanted. Therefore, general guidelines are difficult to formulate, and each patient should get individualised guidance from his personal physician (see also Chapter 10).

Diabetes mellitus

Exercise is an integral part of the treatment of diabetes. But still several precautions are necessary because blood glucose generally falls during exercise, and the long-term effect a of exercise as well as weight loss (which exercise might promote) may increase the sensitivity to the effects of insulin. As discussed later in the chapter on diabetes (Chapter 11), since too high as well as too low a blood glucose level is undesirable, we have to balance the factors which raise the blood glucose with those which lower it on an hour-to-hour basis. Exercise is generally a glucose-lowering procedure (except high-intensity brief exercises like a sprint, which raise blood glucose, and should not be done by those who have diabetes). Therefore, one should not exercise when the effect of insulin or oral drugs is at its peak. Secondly, a sugary snack should be taken about half an hour before the exercise. Thirdly, one should watch out for symptoms of low blood glucose (hypoglycemia). If any such symptoms appear, exercise should be stopped, and sugar or a sweat snack taken. If the person is on insulin, as a general rule, the dose of insulin may be reduced by twenty per cent (i.e. reduced to eighty per cent of the existing dose) at the beginning of the exercise programme. Finer adjustments can be made later depending on the response to exercise. What needs to be emphasised the most in diabetes is consistency. The amount, type and timing of food, drugs and exercise should be constant from day to day and kept at a level which keeps the blood glucose within the desirable range. If any change becomes necessary, a corresponding change should be made in a balancing factor along with observing greater vigilance.

As a general rule, one should not exercise when in a diabetic condition, if the blood glucose level is above 250 mg/dL. An important precaution in those on insulin is not to inject insulin over the exercising muscles: it may be injected in the abdominal fat. Since exercising muscles receive a high blood flow, insulin injected near these muscles enters the bloodstream fast and may bring down the blood glucose to dangerously low levels.

Chronic renal failure

If a person having a kidney disease is on dialysis, exercise should be avoided on the days on which dialysis is to be done. These persons should also avoid intense stretches because tendons have a tendency to rupture in chronic renal failure.

Chronic arthritis

Those having arthritis should spend, even in a yoga session, relatively more time on repetitive exercises (loosening and strengthening exercises) than on steady stretches. If they are on steroids, they should avoid violent movements and falls because steroids induce osteoporosis and increase the risk of getting fractures. If movements are very painful, it might be helpful to concentrate on exercises assisted by gravity or in which gravity is eliminated. For the same reason, exercising in a swimming pool is more comfortable. It also helps to avoid cold exposure, not only during exercise, but even otherwise. As in lung diseases, in arthritis too, one should maintain a strict seven-days-a-week exercise schedule.

Old age

Although old age is not a disease, physical fitness is invariably compromised by age. All the same, it is important for the elderly to exercise in order to remain mobile and functionally independent.

In old age, the warm-up and cooling-down process should be longer, and the intensity of exercise milder than in youth. The weekly increase in intensity of the exercise regime should also be more gradual. Running should be avoided: brisk walking is enough. Running may occasionally trigger a heart attack, and is also likely to cause a sprain or muscle pull which will compel the person to give up exercise for at least a week. The person should also avoid walking on a hilly terrain for the same reason.

During yoga, the elderly should concentrate on asanas which are done in the sitting or lying down posture. If a few postures in the standing posture also have to be done, they may be done with the support of a wall. Inverted postures should be avoided altogether.

Loneliness is a major problem in old age. Therefore exercising in company helps combine exercise with socialising: a highly recommended two-in-one. Walking with a few companions, or joining a group that meets in a park for yogasana and laughter sessions is a healthy practice. Laughter is as important for staying healthy as exercise.

In spite of knowing that exercise is good for health, not many people consciously incorporate it in their daily routine. The commonest excuse for the lapse is that there is no time. First, there is always time for something in which we are interested, something which we consider really important. Secondly, exercise is, in the long run, not at all time-consuming. It improves our efficiency during the rest of the day. It saves the days lost due to illness. It saves the time we spend in hospitals waiting for doctors and getting x-rays and blood tests done. Finally, physical activity can be incorporated in our daily life in ways other than through a formal exercise programme. We can walk to work, at least part of the way. We can use the stairs instead of the lift. One can play with one's grandchild and walk the dog. We can dust the furniture and water the plants. Although adding a structured exercise programme would be better, even these activities are better than none at all.

Frequently Asked Questions

1. *Should underweight persons, who wish to gain weight, exercise?*

   Yes, they should. Exercise is not meant only for losing weight. It has several benefits quite independent of its effects on body weight. Therefore an underweight person should eat well *and* exercise. Paradoxically, this might also help in gaining weight because first, exercise stimulates appetite; and second, exercise promotes muscular development. It is much better to put on weight in the form of muscles rather than fat.

   In addition to a general exercise programme, underweight persons might also find it helpful to practise *chandra anuloma-viloma pranayama* (left nostril breathing): twenty-seven rounds, four times a day. It is said to reduce the metabolic rate (energy expenditure), which should help gain weight.

2. *Is it possible to exercise in the office?*

   It is not only possible, but desirable. If your job involves sitting all the time, find an excuse to stand or walk a little once in an hour or so. For example, you may stand and talk on the phone, walk to the door to receive or see off a visitor, or walk to a colleague next door instead to giving him a call. Second, sedentary jobs also usually keep the neck bent forward. Go through a round of neck exercises (including bending the neck backwards) a few times during office hours to neutralise the continuous posture. Some stretches can also be performed while sitting in the chair. A relaxation technique which can be practised in a chair has been devised by Swami Vivekananda Kendra, Bangalore. Called the instant relaxation technique (IRT), it involves tightening all parts of the body (by contracting the muscles) one by one till the whole body is in a state of maximal tension. The tension is maintained for about five seconds, and then the body is suddenly relaxed completely – not unlike puncturing an inflated balloon.

3. *Is it appropriate to count the pulse for only 10-15 seconds?*

There is no doubt that the count is more accurate if the pulse is counted for at least a full minute: the eminent cardiologist, the late Professor Sujoy B. Roy, taught us that the pulse should be counted for three minutes, and the count divided by three to get the heart rate per minute. But in this chapter, it has been recommended that the pulse be counted for only 10-15 seconds because the context demands it. We want to gauge the intensity of the exercise, for which the proper indicator is the heart rate *during* the exercise. But we measure the heart rate *after* (although immediately after) the exercise. The heart rate starts coming down so rapidly after the exercise that to get close to the heart rate during the exercise, it is better to depend on the count within 10-15 seconds of stopping the exercise.

4. *Can exercise also suppress immunity under some circumstances?*

In general, as mentioned earlier, regular exercise enhances the immunity of the body to various diseases. But it has been found that a single bout of severe and prolonged exercise, such as long distance running, is followed by depressed immunity for about a day. The body recovers from the immunosuppression spontaneously. But it is this temporary immunosuppression which is responsible for the attacks of common cold which follow bouts of intense exercise rather frequently. Further, if intense exercise becomes a daily event, as in professional athletes, it could depress the immunity for longer periods. This discussion leads to two corollaries:

a. Those who wish to exercise only to stay healthy should avoid very strenuous exercise, and
b. Professional athletes should take two precautions. First, they should increase their dietary intake of immunoenhancing antioxidants and phytochemicals.[6] Secondly, when they are recovering from strenuous exercise, they should avoid additional stressors which might depress the immunity. These stressors include dieting, inadequate sleep, and mental stress.

5. *Is an after-dinner walk a healthy practice?*

   Strictly speaking, exercise should be avoided after *any* meal. The reason is that after a meal, the stomach and intestines work hard, and therefore need blood. We do not have to send them more blood: the body has in-built mechanisms for increasing the blood flow to the gut after meals. In the same way, during exercise, blood flow to the exercising muscles increases. Pumping extra blood to two major systems of the body simultaneously means hard work for the heart. That is why exercise should be avoided after meals.

   However, if after-dinner is the only time available for physical activity, then it is better not to lose the opportunity. For many, an after-dinner walk is more than a walk. It is also time for talking to family and friends. Therefore, the practice may be continued, taking care that the walk is *not* brisk. But for those having coronary heart diseases, even a slow leisurely walk should be avoided after any meal.

6. *Does exercise in cold or hot weather need any special precautions?*

   Yes, it does, because both cold and heat impose additional

---

[6] 'Phytochemicals' is a fancy term for some chemicals found in plants. Adequate intake of these chemicals can be ensured by taking enough of fruits and vegetables (about 5 helpings of about 100 g each every day), and by taking spices in moderation.

load on the heart. Therefore those having coronary heart diseases should particularly avoid exercising in extremes of weather. In hot weather, losing the extra heat generated by exercise may also become a problem. It may also become difficult to promptly replace all the water and salts lost through sweating. Therefore in extremes of weather, indoor exercises are preferable, specially for the ill and the elderly.

7. *Does exercise at a hill station need special care?*

Yes, it does because the atmospheric pressure at hill stations is lower than in the plains. Lower atmospheric pressure reduces the availability of oxygen. Therefore the lungs have to work harder at hill stations. Since the oxygen requirement is higher during exercise, a person grows breathless during exercise more easily at high altitude than in the plains. This is particularly important for those having a respiratory problem or a coronary heart disease. When persons go to a hill station, they might have to reduce the intensity of exercise to a level below that which they are usually accustomed to while in the plains in order to stay within safe and comfortable limits.

6

Sweet Dreams

To sleep well one must learn how to sleep.
THE MOTHER
(of Sri Aurobindo Ashram)

It is one of the paradoxes of modern times that in spite of all the time-saving gadgets available to us, we do not have time even to sleep. Mankind, in general, is sleeping rather poorly in today's world. Sleep is as much a part of the lifestyle as eating or exercise. And, evidence is now available indicating that inadequate sleep is one of the contributors to lifestyle diseases.

UNDERSTANDING SLEEP

When a person goes to bed, his sleep is rather light to start with. The sleep deepens progressively and soon the person is in deep dreamless sleep. After a couple of hours of deep dreamless sleep, the sleep begins to get lighter, and the person starts dreaming. The state of dream sleep is also called rapid eye movement (REM) sleep because eyeballs show to-and-fro movements during this phase of sleep: the eyes possibly chase the objects of the dreams. During the state of REM sleep, it is easy to wake a person up, and if we do so, the person is able to narrate the dream. However, we generally do not wake up during the dream. We go through 4-6 cycles of dreamless sleep alternating with dream sleep every night. But since we do not wake up during the dreams, we do not remember them.

Although the state of dreamless sleep alternates with the state of dream sleep throughout the night, the duration of the former is longer, and that of the latter shorter during the initial part. The result is that most of the dreamless sleep occurs during the first half of the night, and most of the dream sleep occurs during the second. Further, the architecture of sleep changes with age. As we get older, the relative time spent in the state of dreamless sleep gets longer, but much of it is not deep. The relative time spent in the state of dream sleep is naturally shorter in the elderly. Further, the pattern of sleep tends to become biphasic: the elderly sleep a little less at night, and compensate for it by sleeping an hour or two during the afternoon. In short, an old person sleeps twice a day, and spends most of the sleep time in a state of shallow dreamless sleep, and a little time in a state of dream sleep (which is also shallow). That is why it is easier to wake up an elderly person than a young person.

The two types of sleep – dreamless and dream sleep – seem to have different functions. Dreamless sleep restores, rejuvenates and refreshes us. Since most of the dreamless sleep occurs in the first half of the night, a person may feel quite fresh even after sleeping for only 4-5 hours. The functions of dream sleep are less clear. In adults, its principal function seems to be consolidation of memory. Anything new that we learn is first stored only for a short period. It becomes a part of long-term memory only after consolidation, which occurs during the state of REM sleep. That is why anything learnt shortly before bedtime is remembered better.

How much sleep do we need?

Most healthy adults need 7-8 hours of sleep. Further, studies have shown that sleeping less than six hours or more than nine hours is associated with adverse effects. All these observations indicate that, on an average, an adult needs 7-8 hours of sleep daily; eight hours is probably safer than seven. However, there is variation in sleep requirements: some need only five hours, while others may need nine hours. The best estimate of the sleep requirement of an individual is the amount of sleep which gives him no symptoms of inadequate sleep.

Sleep during illness

A person generally needs more sleep during an illness. The additional need is easily met because the person feels more sleepy. This happens because some of the chemicals released as a part of the immune response to an illness induce sleep, in addition to their other roles in defense and healing.[1] The moral of the story is that one should not fight the urge to sleep (or the fever, unless it goes above 102°F). We should just sit back, relax and appreciate nature for letting relatively few chemicals do everything that is good for us.

THE EFFECTS OF INADEQUATE SLEEP

If a person has not had enough sleep for a day or two, he is likely to show some of the following effects:

1. Tiredness
2. Difficulty in concentrating, memory disturbances, and poor mental performance.
3. Irritability, frustration, anger and anxiety.
4. High blood pressure.

---

[1] The best known chemical of this type is interleukin-1 (IL-1). Besides inducing sleep, IL-1 also induces fever. The higher body temperature also seems to help in recovery from illness.

5. Increased hunger, and a craving for high carbohydrate and energy-dense foods (eg fried foods).
6. A feeling of pins and needles, or a tingling sensation in the limbs
7. Feeling too cold when others are feeling quite all right.
8. Sleepiness during the day. If the sleep deprivation is severe, sleepiness while driving might lead to an accident.

Some of these effects are all too familiar, and quite expected in terms of common sense. However, some of the effects are such that even doctors are not very conscious of the link. For example, if a patient complains of 'pins and needles' they are more likely to prescribe a cocktail of vitamins B_1, B_6 and B_{12} rather than investigate if the patient is sleeping well.

Effects of chronic sleep deprivation

If sleep deprivation is only for a day or two, the person incurs a sleep debt, and pays it off by sleeping a few extra hours and the ill-effects are reversed. But if sleep deprivation is chronic, it cannot be balanced. The result is a variety of adverse effects listed below:

1. Impaired immunity, leading to frequent infections such as a common cold.
2. Weight gain, which is at least partly due to the hunger induced by sleep deprivation.
3. The triad of diabetes, hypertension and coronary heart disease.
4. Depression and other manifestations of mental stress.

VOLUNTARY SLEEP RESTRICTION

There is a global trend towards cutting down on sleep time. According to a recent poll conducted by the market research firm AC Nielsen, the Japanese are the most sleep-deprived people in the world today. In terms of bedtime, the Portuguese top the list, with seventy-five per cent going to bed after midnight. We Indians do a lot better: only twenty-nine per cent go to bed after midnight, but sixty-one per cent of us sleep less than seven hours a day because we get up rather early by world standards. Being an internet survey, it is likely to be biased, but that is no reason for complacency. The fact is that many Indians are now sleeping less than they should.

The question arises as to why so many people are cutting down on one of the pleasant necessities of life which is available to all free of cost. A major factor is too much work to do, which is the price we pay to maintain a good standard of living. However, along with the work, we do not want to neglect many other important and not-so-important things as well, which makes matters worse so far as sleep is concerned. We want to spend time with the family, we do not want to miss out on parties, and we want to watch some serials on TV and also some movies on DVDs. Watching TV or a movie at home might seem like wonderful multi-tasking – information, entertainment, 'relaxation', and spending time with the family – all in one. And, if there is a member of the family who would much rather sleep than watch TV or participate in family gossip, she dare not be the odd-one-out, specially if she happens to be the daughter-in-law. Worse still, when the family goes to bed and the infant wakes up for a midnight meal, the brunt of that too has to be borne, by and large, by the poor daughter-in-law! Her husband, even if he is willing to help, might be spared because he is by then busy with homework that he has brought from office. Evening is also the time to catch up with friends by giving them a call or by e-mailing. And, once you are on the net, one may just surf from one thing to the other without realising how much time has passed. The telephone and internet become even more tempting at night because they may cost less during these hours. Finally, if this goes on for a few years, and one finds everybody else also doing the same, going to bed unnaturally late seems like the most natural thing to do! In short, sleeping late becomes a habit.

It may still be possible to sleep enough if one could get up late.[2] But even that becomes difficult because apart from the in-built body rhythms waking us up at the 'normal' time, there are other factors to contend with. The school bus comes at 7 am, the traffic on the roads get unbearable after 8 am, the wife has to be dropped at 9 am, the office begins at 10 am, and so on.

What can we do about it?

Many of the points made above might strike you as 'so true' because you can identify with them. But describing and analysing the situation does not solve the problem. Is there something we can do about it?

In general, there is no problem about which nothing can be done. What is required is the will, and the way will reveal itself. To generate the will, the priorities need to be fixed. If we consider sleep important, time will somehow be found. After all, the day has twenty-four hours, of which we may stay awake for sixteen hours, or stretch these hours to eighteen at the expense of sleep. First, are there absolutely no activities less important than sleep, on which we spend up to two hours during the day? Second, can we not do some of the daytime activities more efficiently and thereby save time? Third, can our efficiency not be improved by sleeping longer! Fourth, don't we pay back the time saved by sleeping less many times over a few years later by spending time in hospitals? Finally, by falling sick due to lack of sleep, don't we harm the very family for whose sake we apparently cut down on sleep?

These are simple questions, to which the answers are obvious. But in today's hectic lifestyle, we don't have even the time to pause

---

[2] Sleeping late and getting up late makes sleep out of phase with other daily rhythms of the body, and is therefore not as refreshing as 'normal' (early-to-bed and early-to-rise) sleep.

and ask these questions. What is required is to basically slow down a bit, pause, reflect, reset priorities, and reschedule activities a bit to add two hours to sleep – just two hours is generally the difference between the actual and ideal sleep time. Further, the sleep itself can be made more efficient so that we get more rest in less time. Of this, we shall learn a little later in the chapter.

GOSSIP

To gossip about what somebody is doing or not doing is wrong. To listen to such gossip is wrong. To verify if such gossip is true is wrong. To retaliate in words against a false gossip is wrong.

The whole affair is a very bad way of wasting one's time and lowering one's consciousness.

THE MOTHER
(of Sri Aurobindo Ashram)

SLEEPLESSNESS

Inadequate sleep is not necessarily due to spending less time in bed: it may be because of difficulty in either falling asleep, or staying asleep. Such disorders, collectively called insomnia, may or may not be associated with voluntary sleep restriction. Let us first see how insomnia and voluntary sleep restriction may be interrelated. Suppose a person cuts down on sleeping time due to work pressure. The work may be so much that it remains unfinished in spite of going to bed late. When the person finally does go to bed, he starts worrying about the unfinished work. The worry makes it difficult for him to fall asleep. Thus he remains awake while lying down in the bed. He tries hard to sleep, which makes falling asleep even harder!

However, most people having insomnia spend more than enough time in bed but still fail to get enough sleep. Insomnia is generally due to mental stress: unfinished work is only one of the causes of stress; there could be many more. Insomnia may also be due to inadequate physical activity during the day. But too much physical activity or mental excitement just before bedtime also makes it difficult for one to fall asleep. Sleeping at the wrong time may also be difficult even if one needs sleep badly. For example, it may be difficult to sleep during the day even if one has been awake the whole night. Another cause of insomnia may be tea or coffee taken before bedtime. Some persons are so sensitive to caffeine that taking these drinks even three hours before bedtime might make it difficult for them to fall asleep.

Alcohol selectively suppresses REM sleep. Therefore, after an evening drinking alcohol, REM sleep is suppressed during the first half of the night. To compensate for it, there is an excess of REM sleep in the second half of the night. Since REM sleep is accompanied by dreams, the person may wake up repeatedly in the second half of the night with vivid dreams, and sometimes nightmares.

Sleep apnea

Apnea means the stoppage of breathing. Some persons habitually get recurrent stoppage of breathing during sleep. The mechanism of the stoppage is similar to that of snoring. When a person sleeps, all the muscles of the body are relaxed. These muscles include muscles that keep the airways properly open. When these muscles relax, the airways may become narrow, leading to snoring. In extreme cases, snoring may be followed by the throat getting completely blocked leading to sleep apnea. However, this apnea cannot last very long. In such situations, the body has mechanisms which create a strong urge to breathe. These mechanisms also generally make the person very restless, and he wakes up. However, when the person falls asleep again, the musculature relaxes and he may get sleep apnea. The apnea wakes up the person, and he starts breathing. The alternation may continue: the person can either breathe or sleep, and he ends up doing both rather poorly. The cycle of apnea and awakening may repeat itself hundreds of times in one night. Thus sleep apnea, apart from being a bit scary, also leads to sleep deprivation and its adverse effects, specially daytime sleepiness. Sleep apnea is typically a problem during middle age, and is commonly associated with obesity. All obese persons do not get sleep apnea; but about half of the persons who get sleep apnea are obese. Sleep apnea is common after drinking in the evening, and is more dangerous if the person is lying down flat on the back. Therefore, the simplest measures one may adopt by way of treatment are to avoid alcohol in the evening, lose some weight if the person is overweight, and to sleep lying on the side. If these do not help, a specialist should be consulted.

TREATING SLEEP DEFICIT

Much of the discussion that follows is currently called 'sleep hygiene'. Sleep hygiene is a component of a life lived with moderation and wisdom, and is therefore good for all – for those who sleep well, and those who do not, be it due to voluntary restriction or due to a sleep disorder.

Before a person starts getting concerned about not sleeping enough, it is also good to remember that people differ in their sleep requirement. If a person sleeps only 5-6 hours every night, but during the day does not feel sleepy, is not irritable or restless, and is able to concentrate properly on his work without drinking tea or coffee, then possibly that is all the sleep he needs. He is just one of those lucky persons who need less sleep, and the best way he can express his gratitude to God for this gift is by being more productive.

If a person has genuine difficulty in falling asleep, or staying asleep, it should be taken as a message. Through this difficulty, his body is telling him about some disharmony in life – bodily neglect, emotional overload, mental confusion, or disorganised consciousness. He should heed the message, and restore harmony using the principles of yoga. Maybe he needs to rein in the unreasonable demands of his ego, or take a more charitable view of the faults of his fellow beings, or accept life's vicissitudes with equanimity born of surrender to the divine will and wisdom. Once harmony returns to his life, sleep will take care of itself.

Spending the day well

A day spent well paves the way for a good night's sleep, just as a good night's sleep prepares us for a pleasant day. Spend the day peacefully and productively. Manage your time well. Don't leave too many loose ends. Avoid inefficiency and needless gossip.

Have a schedule which is in tune with nature, specially your nature. Do not try to get up too early, or stay in bed too long, or to sleep too early in the evening. However, the timings of the body rhythms differ from person to person. Find out yours, and try to have a schedule which is in tune with your body rhythms.

Stay physically active. Early morning any kind of physical activity (walking, jogging, or yogic exercises) is good for health, but has no direct effect on the tendency to sleep at night. Moderate physical activity late in the afternoon or early in the evening facilitates falling asleep at night. Strenuous physical activity within three hours before bedtime makes it difficult for one to fall asleep.

If you take an afternoon nap, it should be just about one hour, not much longer. Have an early dinner: try to have at least an hour's gap between dinner and bedtime. Further, the dinner should not be heavy.

Avoid smoking and tobacco products: nicotine tends to keep a person awake. Avoid tea and coffee late in the evening: if you are particularly sensitive to caffeine, do not take tea or coffee within six hours of bedtime. Do not take alcohol within two hours before bedtime for undisturbed sleep. The ideal, of course, is to avoid all these products altogether.

Bedtime rituals

It is specially important that at least an hour, preferably two hours, immediately preceding bedtime should be spent in peaceful and relaxing activities. Excitement and strenuous physical activity release adrenaline. Adrenaline once released cannot be called back, and adrenaline keeps a person awake. The only solution then is to let the body metabolise the adrenaline and bring its level down, and that takes a couple of hours. What it means in practical terms is to avoid books and movies with blood-curdling plots or loud and fast music near bedtime. Even long and engaging phone calls should be avoided. Also, avoid taking too much of fluids close to bedtime to avoid the need for getting up in the middle of the night for emptying the bladder. However, a cup of hot milk or herbal 'tea' (without the herb called tea!) close to bedtime facilitates sleepiness. After the drink, brush your teeth, wash your feet, empty the bladder, and settle down with a pleasant book, some soothing music, or a peaceful TV programme. Some people find a warm water bath a helpful bedtime ritual. Among the yogic practices, alternate nostril breathing (*nadi shuddhi pranayama*) promotes a particularly peaceful feeling which is good preparation for falling asleep.

By now you might be cursing me for creating a romantic picture of the hour before bedtime. You might be thinking 'It is easy for him to write all this. What does he know of my life with two telephones ringing and a baby wailing simultaneously near bedtime'? The reason why this rather unrealistic picture has been painted is that unless we know the ideal, we cannot even move towards it. Secondly, if a person has genuine difficulty falling asleep, he should be prepared to put in some effort to create conditions conducive to sleep. Thirdly, the human body has so much resilience that fortunately, most of us can get away with a lot of indiscretion. Finally, for falling asleep, what matters more than any bedtime ritual is probably the combination of hard work and a clear conscience.

How to sleep

There is no way a person can force himself to fall asleep: the person just slips into sleep – that is why it is called 'falling' asleep. Therefore there is no set method by which a person may be guaranteed to go to sleep within a fixed period of time. Yet, there are ways by which conditions conducive to sleep might be created. These conditions make it highly probable that the person will fall asleep within a short time.

A basic requirement for promoting sleep is to reduce sensory stimuli. To achieve this, the bedroom should be dark, quiet, neither too cold nor too hot, and the bed should be comfortable. One may achieve silence outside, but if there is noise within, sleeping becomes difficult. Noise within arises from worries, anxieties, and thoughts about events during the day – highly positive as well as highly negative events can both be equally noisy.[3] Assure yourself that first, worrying does not solve any problems; second, nothing will change overnight; third, pray that the next day God guides you towards resolution of the issue. Treat your pillow as the lap of the god/goddess/guru towards whom you have a sense of devotion. Feel the comfort and the sense of security in the pillow which a child experiences in a mother's lap. Leave all your cares to the one you adore, at least for the night, and trust him/her to see you through the problem in his/her way and in his/her time. Regarding the exciting events of the day which are keeping you awake, review the day and sort out the events into those which you are proud of, and those which you have reason to be ashamed of. For the ones you are proud of, be grateful for the divine grace which made them possible. For those you are ashamed of, ask the Divine for forgiveness, and resolve to do better in similar circumstances next time. That is the constructive

---

[3] As Hans Selye, the father of physiology of stress said, a passionate kiss can be as stressful as a painful blow.

way of dealing with mistakes. It does not pay to carry the heavy burden of guilt all the time. These exercises, carried out sincerely for their own sake, and not only for the sake of sleep, will relax your mind.

Next, relax your body completely, as during *shavasana*. When your body is completely relaxed, you get a feeling as though you are sinking into the bed every time you breathe out. This is what is generally referred to as deep relaxation.[4] When the body and mind are totally relaxed, sleep comes by easily. In fact, most people fall asleep even before completing the process, although the process can be completed in less than five minutes.

If you have achieved a state of deep relaxation, and have not yet fallen asleep, it is in a way a happy situation. You now have an opportunity to meditate. While continuing to lie down in a state deep relaxation, start a slow, silent chanting of the sound which you normally use in meditation. Synchronise the chanting with breathing (Chapter 2). Within a few minutes, you will fall asleep.

The above process is not meant only for those who have difficulty falling asleep. It is the right way to fall asleep for everybody, because it ensures not just sleep, but the right kind of sleep. A person who goes to bed exhausted, or starts dozing off while reading a thriller, might instantly fall asleep. But this will be a disturbed kind of sleep, a sleep interrupted by bad dreams, even nightmares. The 'three ways' of falling asleep have been shown in Fig. 6.1.

What should one do if one is unable to sleep?

It is quite possible that in spite of doing everything right, once in a while you will find it difficult to fall asleep. It is understood

---

[4] It is not essential to relax the mind before relaxing the body. You may relax the body before relaxing the mind, or relax both simultaneously.

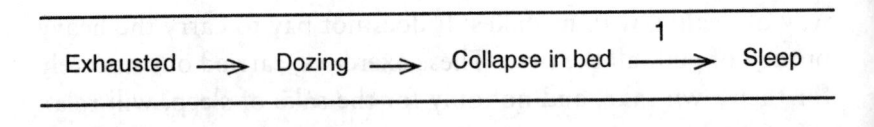

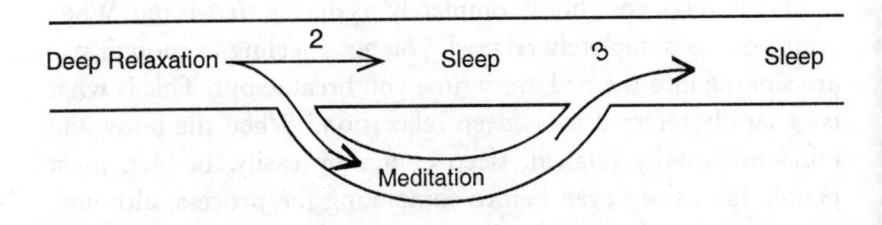

```
Exhausted  →  Dozing  →  Collapse in bed  →¹  Sleep


Deep Relaxation  →²  Sleep  →³  Sleep
                ↘         ↗
                  Meditation
```

Fig. 6.1. Three routes to sleep (1-3). Route 1 is bad: it leads to poor quality disturbed sleep. Route 2 is satisfactory, but route 3 gives the best quality sleep.

that if you have not fallen asleep while achieving a state of deep relaxation, you would start meditating. Suppose you have been meditating for twenty to twenty-five minutes, and are still wide awake, it is not wise to get anxious, and to look at the clock again and again. The best thing to do in this situation is to get up, get out of bed, and start doing something. You may read, do some light chore (like tidying up a congested drawer), or do something serious that needs to get done. It is quite possible that an important pending job is what is keeping you awake. The satisfaction you will get when it gets done will send you to sleep. In short, if you cannot sleep, it is better to be fully awake instead of tossing and turning in bed, and getting more anxious with every passing hour. After you have done something interesting for an hour or two, you may try sleeping again. You may practice five-ten rounds of *nadi shuddhi pranayama* (alternate nostril breathing) before lying down. Lie down, go into a state of deep relaxation, and start meditating, and hope for the best.

Occasional sleep deprivation has neither long-term nor any serious short-term implications. It is surprising but true that if you have a busy day following a sleepless night, you are able to go through the day quite efficiently: it is only towards the evening that you start feeling more sleepy than usual. Some of the things that should or should not be done when you are unable to sleep at night have been summarised in Table 6.1.

Table 6.1. DOS AND DON'TS WHEN UNABLE TO SLEEP

Dos	Don'ts
Get up and do something interesting.	Don't keep tossing and turning in bed.
Take it easy: insomnia is neither a crime nor the end of the world.	Don't get anxious, don't try hard to sleep, don't look at the clock every half an hour.
Rest assured that even if you do not sleep well tonight, you can go through the day efficiently. Your performance in a crucial meeting, or in your lecture, can still be brilliant.	Don't keep thinking that if I do not sleep within the next one hour, the next day is ruined.

How to wake up

There is a popular misconception that sound sleep means that a person should sleep continuously for 7-8 hours without waking up even once. The fact is that we all wake up briefly several times during the night, quickly go to sleep again, and by the morning do not even remember that we had woken up. A person practising yoga does everything consciously, including sleeping. Therefore, such a person not only wakes up several times during the night, but even remembers that he had woken up. Further, he uses each awakening to go into a state of deep relaxation, meditate, and slip into sleep – all this while continuing to lie down. The process makes sleep more peaceful and improves the quality of sleep as a whole, including that of the dreams. As the Mother (of Sri Aurobindo Ashram) puts it, sleep should be cut into slices. The first slice is about three hours long. After that, each slice is about one hour. After about five slices, that is, after 7-8 hours of sleep, one feels fully rested, and it is time to get up. To keep lying in bed beyond this point is laziness. Once the Mother was asked why it was so difficult to get up in the morning. She replied something to the effect that she could not understand the question. Once you are awake, what is difficult about getting up, she asked. It is true that unless a person is paralysed, there should be no difficulty in getting up. The difficulty is due to laziness. Laziness comes from treating the bed as a warm and comfortable place where we need not work. To avoid such laziness, two things are important. First, we should understand that the bed is only a 'recharge station': a place where we recharge our batteries so that we are ready for yet another day's work. Secondly, we should love our work, treating it as an opportunity to offer something to the Divine. If these two requirements are met, there will be no room for laziness.

However, it does not mean that as soon as we are awake, we should jump out of bed. Getting up should also be, like everything else, a peaceful and conscious process. For example, one may gently sit up in bed, keeping the eyes closed. One should thank God for yet another day to work for Him, and to improve as a person. Then one may meditate for a few minutes, and resolve to maintain a meditative poise throughout the day. Then one may open the eyes with a few blinks, and get down from the bed.[5]

If a person has insomnia, after getting out of bed, one of the first things he should do is to fill up the sleep diary. A sleep diary is a daily record of bedtime, waking up time, duration of sleep,

---

[5] Such a peaceful transition from waking up to getting up, apart from being good in itself, will also prevent any fall in blood pressure on standing up. The elderly are particularly prone to such a drop in blood pressure, and as a result might fall upon standing. As an added precaution, the elderly may take some support from a wall, a door handle, or any other suitable object while getting down from the bed.

quality of sleep, and the state of well-being at the time of waking up, i.e. fresh and active, or dull and lazy. The diary provides a feedback to the person, and is a source of encouragement as the person observes an overall improvement week after week. However, if a person does everything mentioned in this chapter, he will neither have insomnia nor need a sleep diary.

A few additional don'ts for the sleep-deprived

Do not sleep for too long, even if you can afford to get up late. Also, do not go to bed too early in an effort to make up for lost sleep. In short, observe proper timings in tune with the day-night rhythm of nature.

Do not try to sleep till late in the morning on weekends. An hour or two extra may be fine, but do not stay in bed, asleep or awake, till late in the morning just because you can afford to.

Finally, do not use sleeping pills for at least three reasons. First, they induce dependence. After some time, it becomes difficult to sleep without the pill. And, with time, the dose required to fall asleep tends to go up. Secondly, pills have side effects. Finally, pills do not induce normal sleep. They suppress deep dreamless sleep as well as dream sleep. The result is that the person is in a state of shallow dreamless sleep most of the times. Therefore, although the duration of the sleep under the influence of sleeping pills may be normal, the person does not get up fresh and energetic. Sleeping pills have a place only for occasional use in times be acute stress. They should not be used for habitual or chronic sleeplessness.

VIOLATING NATURAL RHYTHMS

Life has evolved in such a way as to be adapted to the twenty-four-hour cycle of day and night. Several rhythms in the human body have a 24-hour cycle: sleep-wakefulness is only one of them. Some of the other 24-hour rhythms are the hormonal rhythms (specially that of cortisol, the 'stress hormone'), temperature rhythm and immunity rhythm. Further, all these rhythms are normally linked to light and darkness. The fluctuations in these functions over the 24-hour period are such that it is conducive to one's well-being. For example, it is easier to work in a bright light, and rest when it is dark. Similarly, stress is more likely to occur soon after we are awake, and therefore the hormone which is useful in stressful situations should have a higher level at waking-up time. Thus the rise in cortisol coincides with the waking-up time. If we disturb the synchronisation of these rhythms, the body suffers. For example, if we sleep late and get up late, even if the duration of sleep is adequate, the quality is poor, and we feel tired during the day. This happens because we have slept during the wrong time while all the other rhythms stayed on the correct schedule. We do not have much control over biological rhythms other than sleep. Therefore, all we can do for optimum body functions is to keep our sleep timings as much as possible, in tune with nature. We violate body rhythms most violently white working night shifts and travelling.

Shift work

It is because various body rhythms are tied up with one another that a person who does a night shift finds it difficult to sleep during the day even if he has the time. If a person works at night for several days in a row, he can change all his body rhythms by working at night in bright light, and during the day, making the bedroom as dark as possible. When his rhythms adapt to the new light-dark cycle, he gets used to night shifts. However, this cannot be done if the night shift is only once or twice a week. Therefore, it is better to have night duty everyday for a few weeks, and then day duty everyday for a few weeks, than to have just one or two night duties a week throughout the year. However, it is often difficult to arrange the ideal schedule in real life situations. That is why those who work in shifts are prone to get stress-related disorders, particularly high blood pressure, coronary heart disease, and peptic ulcer.

Jet lag

Jet lag is the unpleasant feeling of tiredness, restlessness and mental confusion many people experience when they travel a long distance by air. A plane can transport us quickly to a place where it is day, while it is night at the place from where we started. At the end of the journey, the body rhythms, still tied up to the light-dark cycle of the place from where we started, create the symptoms of jet lag. The rhythms adapt to the light-dark cycle of the new place in a few days, and the symptoms disappear. In order to hasten this adaptation to the new place, it is best to spend as much time as possible in sunlight at the new place. The process can be further hastened by taking a tablet of melatonin (a hormone which is normally released at night) at night. Further, as a preparation for such a journey, one may start making a gradual and progressive shift in the sleep timings towards what they will be like at the new place, a few days before the journey, making the room dark while sleeping, and staying in a brightly lit room when awake.

CLOSING THOUGHTS

Sleeping late and sleeping less, have become a part of modern lifestyle, and are making a significant contribution to lifestyle diseases. A balanced and sensible approach to life should help in improving our sleep along with making our lifestyle healthy in every other respect. Yoga, the best lifestyle ever devised, not only helps us fall asleep easily but also improves the quality of sleep as well as wakefulness. Thus we get more rest from every hour that we spend in bed, and are able to work better and feel better when we are out of bed.

Frequently Asked Questions

1. *Why does a person feel sleepy at 9 pm but wide awake two hours later?*

    This happens because at 9 pm all body rhythms are geared towards sleep. If sleep is somehow resisted at that time, the golden time when everything is synchronised is gone. In terms of ayurveda, after 10 pm a person makes a transition from the *kapha* phase to the *pitta* phase, which is a transition from inactivity to activity. Therefore, staying active beyond 10 pm and sleeping after that leads to disturbed sleep.

2. *Is it all right to use an alarm clock for waking up on time?*

    No, the alarm may go off while one is in a state of deep dreamless sleep or in the middle of a dream, which are not the normal and natural phases for awakening to take place. Further, waking up with an alarm is abrupt, whereas normal awakening is a gradual process. Therefore a person who wakes up with the help of an alarm clock is unlikely to get up refreshed.

7

Don't Worry, Be Happy

Our mental attitudes affect first our susceptibility to disease and then our ability to overcome it.

BERNIE SIEGEL, MD

Stress is a part of life. But undue stress, unproductive stress or unmitigated stress turns into distress. And, the general feeling is that stress levels have gone up within the last few decades. Let us reflect on how it has happened. During the last few centuries, the world has changed at a pace unprecedented in human history. Science and technology have given us time-saving gadgets, means of rapid transport, and almost instantaneous communication. However, the more these 'conveniences' have made life easier, the more it seems to have become difficult. The sources of tension in life have not reduced one bit, the world-wide web notwithstanding. Human nature has not changed, and therefore hatred, jealousy and intrigues continue to plague mankind as much today as in the days of the *Mahabharata*. Further, the proliferation of consumer goods has made man more self-centred, and increased the frustrations due to unfulfilled (and fulfilled!) desires. The association between increasing mental stress and the rising prevalence of several diseases of modern civilisation has compelled man to sit up and take notice of the time-honoured wisdom enshrined in ancient systems such as yoga. While none of these systems can guarantee a life free of stress, they do show a way for acquiring mastery over sources of stress.

EFFECTS OF STRESS ON THE BODY

Anyone who has experienced a dry mouth and pounding heart during stress knows that stress affects the body. The effects of stress on the body evolved quite early in the course of evolution, and are primarily designed to help the animal face the stressful situation better. In order to understand how, let us consider an encounter between a lion and a deer. The lion is overcome by an aggressive impulse, and the deer by fear. These emotions help both animals in intensifying their effort: the lion while it is running to catch the deer, and the deer while it is running to escape. Thus emotional stress intensifies the effort, and improves the chances of success in *both* the animals. Hence stress is useful. Further, success in the stressful situation depends at least partly on the ability to run well. The effects of stress on the body help in running better. While running, the exercising muscles need more blood, more oxygen, and more glucose. Increase in heart rate and increase in the force with which the heart beats helps increase blood flow. More blood carries more oxygen to the muscles. Further, the rate and depth of breathing increase, and the airways open up in stress, helping delivery of more oxygen to the body. In stress, glycogen in the liver and muscles also breaks down to release glucose, thereby making more glucose available to the muscles. Several other effects of stress on the body also help. For example, the pupils of the eye become wide open. As a result, even in dark the animal is able to make the best use of whatever little light is available, and thereby find his way better. In short, stress has effects on the body which are useful in the stressful situation. Hence these effects have survival value.

If the effects of stress on the body are useful, why do they lead to disease in man? To begin with, it needs to be emphasised that they are useful to man as well. Although human beings do not hunt any more, they find it difficult to survive without these mechanisms. But two peculiarities of human life make the same mechanisms harmful under certain conditions. *First*, as compared to animals, human beings have a very good memory, and they make plans for the future. As a result, their stress becomes long-term, or chronic. In animals, stress is based only on the present. For example, in the case of a lion chasing a deer, the stress begins when they spot each other, and ends when the deer has been caught, or when it has become out of reach. But in human beings stress may be due to what happened years ago, or what might go wrong years later! Prolonged stress makes some of the effects of acute stress on the body continuous, and that is harmful. For example, a rise in blood pressure while running is perfectly normal, but it becomes a disease if it is continuous. Our body, like that of animals, is primarily designed to face acute stress, not for coping up with chronic stress. *Secondly*, even in acute stress, human beings often do not have to indulge in physical activity. By and large, the 'civilised' man today neither has to chase his prey, nor has to flee from a predator. When he fights with his fellow beings, he generally confines himself to a verbal attack; only rarely does the attack become physical. Due to absence of physical activity during acute stress, the response may turn harmful. For example, if the muscle and liver glycogen break down to release glucose, but additional glucose does not get utilised (because there are no exercising muscles),

> What has happened to me today and what will happen early on the morrow again? I am not afflicted by such worries. Therefore I live without disease.
> – VASHISHTA DARSHANAM

the glucose remains in blood, thereby raising the blood glucose level. If prolonged stress makes a high blood glucose level almost continuous, it may contribute to diabetes. Similarly, if the heart beats faster and more forcefully, but the blood flow through muscles does not increase (because muscles are not exercising), the heart will have to work harder, and its hard work will raise the blood pressure even more (Fig. 7.1). If chronic stress makes this rise in blood pressure almost continuous, it may lead to hypertension.

The effects of stress are not confined to the heart or liver. How widespread these effects are, and how chronic stress may contribute to a wide variety of diseases will become clearer if we understand how the effects of stress on the body are mediated.

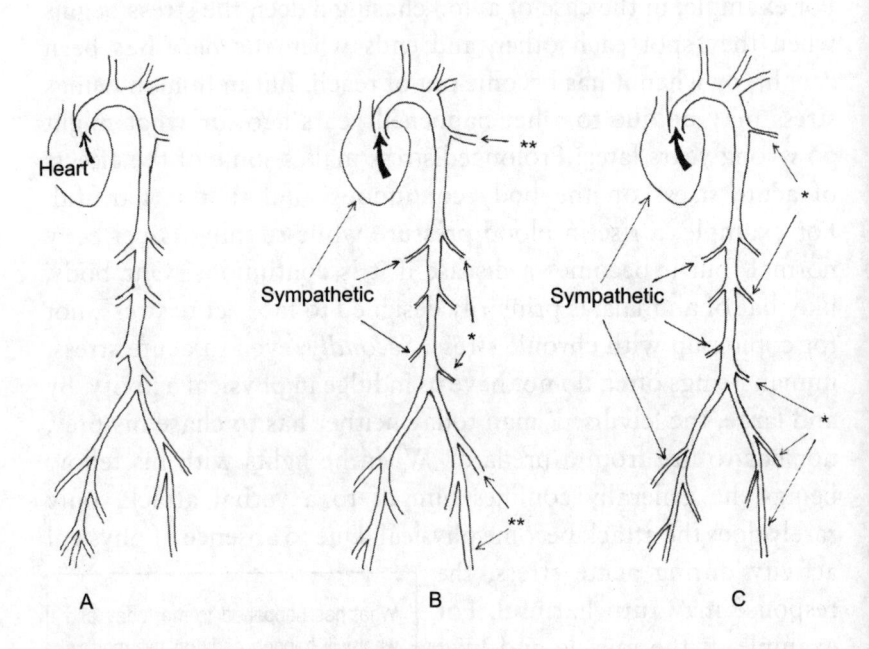

Fig. 7.1. *The mechanism whereby sympathetic activation raises blood pressure.*
A. *A normal resting left ventricle of the heart pumping blood into the arterial tree.*
B. *Sympathetic activation makes the heart beat faster and more forcefully, and constricts the blood vessels (*). However, in exercising muscles, the blood vessels are dilated (**)*
C. *The sympathetic nervous system is activated and blood vessels are constricted (*) everywhere because there are no exercising muscles. Therefore there will be a marked rise in blood pressure.*

How does stress affect the body?

The foundation of stress resides in our thoughts and emotions. One might roughly say that thoughts are associated with the activity of the highest part of the brain, the cerebral cortex. On the other hand, emotions are associated with the activity of another division of the brain, the limbic system. Both the cortex and limbic system channelise their effects during stress to a tiny part of the brain, called the hypothalamus. Hypothalamus is a vital integrating knot which affects at least three systems which have wide-ranging effects on the body (Fig. 7.2). The three systems are autonomic nervous system, endocrine system and immune system.

```
        ┌─────────────────┐
        │ Cerebral cortex │
        └─────────────────┘
              │   ▲
              ▼   │
        ┌─────────────────┐
        │  Limbic system  │
        └─────────────────┘
                │
                ▼
        ┌─────────────────┐
        │  Hypothalamus   │
        └─────────────────┘
          ╱     │     ╲
         ╱   Endocrines  ╲
        ╱       │         ╲
      ANS                Immune
                         system

   ┌──────────────────────────────┐
   │ Effects of Stress on the Body│
   └──────────────────────────────┘
```

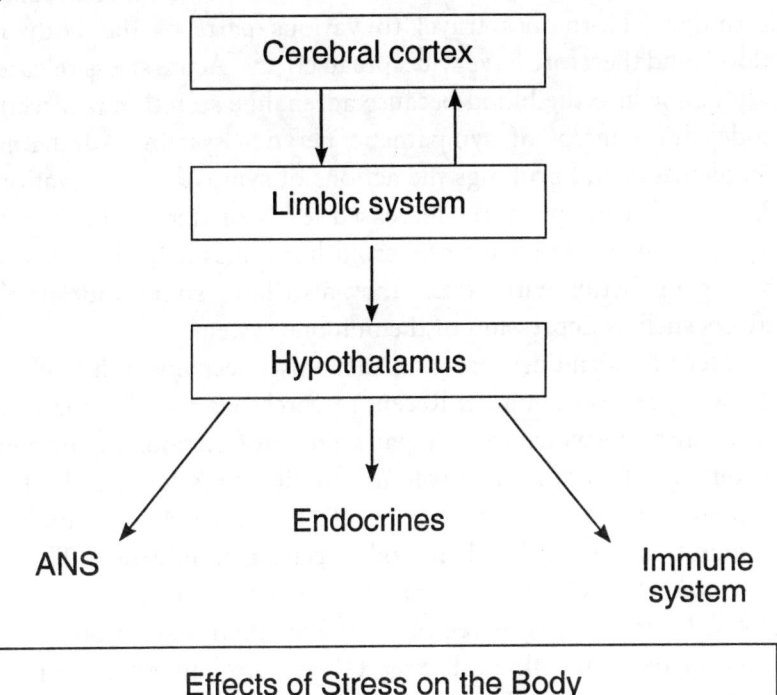

Fig. 7.2. *Effects of stress on the body. ANS, Autonomic nervous system.*

The autonomic nervous system modulates the activity of internal organs of the body such as heart, stomach or urinary bladder. Autonomic system has two subdivisions: sympathetic and parasympathetic. The sympathetic division is more active during stress, and affects the activity of internal organs in a manner that would be helpful in coping up with stress. That is why it is called 'sympathetic': it helps us when we are in trouble. On the other hand, the parasympathetic division is more active when we are at rest and relaxed. Prolonged stress creates a long-term imbalance between sympathetic and parasympathetic activity. The imbalance can predispose us to several diseases associated with stress, such as heart disease, high blood pressure and peptic ulcer.

The endocrine system produces a set of chemicals called hormones. Hormones travel to various parts of the body in blood, and therefore have widespread effects. Acute stress releases adrenaline into the blood because adrenaline secretion is directly under the control of sympathetic nervous system. Adrenaline supplements and prolongs the actions of sympathetic activation. Prolonged stress produces increased levels of steroid hormones. While most of the effects of steroid hormones help the body in coping up better with stress, they also have some undesirable effects such as depression of the immune system.

Steroid hormones are not the only mechanism by which stress depresses immunity. Recent research has revealed multiple mechanisms by which stress impairs immune function. Impairment of immune function has profound implications for health. The immune system protects us from infections. Therefore impaired immunity increases the likelihood of getting an infection. That is why common cold is the commonest when one is under mental stress. Further, allergies (eg bronchial asthma) and autoimmune diseases (eg some thyroid diseases) are also an expression of deranged immunity. Finally, now it is clear that the immune system protects us also against cancer. Thus impaired immunity can increase the risk of cancer as well.

IMPLICATIONS OF THE EFFECTS OF STRESS ON THE BODY

The above discussion makes it clear that prolonged stress can act through various mechanisms to increase the risk of high blood pressure, heart disease, diabetes, peptic ulcer, infections, cancer, allergies and autoimmune diseases. Stress being such a common phenomenon, that is a very depressing thought indeed! A bright implication of these facts, however, is that the reverse of stress, i.e. positive emotions, can do just the opposite. Not only can positive emotions prevent illness, they can even heal an illness. In other words, the disease process initiated by stress is reversible.

Norman Cousins, a perceptive and learned man, but not a doctor, figured out on his own that his serious autoimmune disease was possibly related to a few days of acute stress he had experienced shortly before the onset of his illness. He reasoned that if stress could make him sick, cheerfulness might make him well again. He treated himself with laughter (by watching comedies) and vitamin C, and actually recovered. His book, *Anatomy of an Illness* has now become a classic.

Bernie Siegel, a cancer surgeon, suspected that his patients had some personality traits and traumatic life experiences which might have contributed to their illness. Therefore he started treating his patients with, in addition to the usual medical treatment, psychological support and counselling. He found that this always made the remainder of the life of his patients more tolerable in spite of cancer, and frequently even made the remainder longer. Books documenting his experiences and other studies along the same lines are now available as popular paperbacks.

Dean Ornish, a cardiologist, demonstrated that lifestyle modification, of which stress reduction was a major component, led to a reduction in the blockage of coronary arteries in his patients. This refuted the classical medical teaching that coronary artery disease may at best remain stable, but generally gets worse. Now we know that it can even get better. Dean Ornish's book on his programme for 'reversal' of heart disease is also a popular paperback.[1]

The above discussion brings out two encouraging facts:
(a) Positive emotions can heal a variety of illnesses.
(b) Thousands of patients have got rid of mental stress by changing their attitude to people, events and circumstances, and have thereby achieved healing. If so many have done it, why can't you?

> Establish a greater peace and quietness in your body; that will give you the strength to resist attacks of illness.
>
> — THE MOTHER
> (of Sri Aurobindo Ashram)

GENERAL CAUSES OF STRESS

The general causes of stress may be best summed up in the words of Patanjali:

> Ignorance, ego, likes and dislikes, and clinging to life are the causes of misery.
>
> (*Yoga Sutras*, 2:3)

According to Swami Vivekananda's interpretation of this sutra, ignorance is the basic cause of misery, the rest are the result of ignorance. The ignorance referred to here is not one that can be removed by going to a school or college. Yoga is based on a

---

[1] Here 'reversal' applies to the process by which the disease develops. The process consists of progressive narrowing of coronary blood vessels. 'Reversal' means progressive widening of the blood vessels. If a person's blood vessels are blocked to the extent of 70%, even if they remain blocked 65% after one year, the process has reversed. Thus 'reversal' does not mean that the arteries become completely free of the block.

spiritual worldview. The spiritual worldview gives us knowledge about the nature and purpose of life. As a result we learn to look at people, events and circumstances in light of this knowledge. For example, once we know that all creation is a manifestation of the same Divine, our self-absorption is diminished, and our ego tends to get eliminated. According to Sri Aurobindo, desires starve in the absence of support from the ego. Desires are a fundamental cause of misery, as emphasised by Buddha. Also, being able to visualise the same divine spark in all persons, we start judging people rather charitably. Further, being able to visualise the divine hand behind all happenings improves our cheerful acceptance of events and circumstances. Reduction in self-absorption, acceptance of mortality of the body, and knowledge of immortality of the soul reduce the tendency to cling to life. Thus a sincere cultivation of the yogic attitude can eliminate the sources of stress. Rather, the yogic attitude can induce a state of stable and sustained peace and joy, which is independent of external events and circumstances.

> Most of the difficulties that people have are due to a lack of control over their actions, and their reactions to the actions of others.
>
> — THE MOTHER
> (of Sri Aurobindo Ashram)

STRESS MANAGEMENT

The key to stress management is to develop a clear insight into the problem. To get the insight, it is helpful to ask oneself a few searching questions. Find a quiet corner, relax, and ask yourself these questions during meditation. The sooner you do so, the better, because the more you let stress accumulate, the more difficult the issue might get.

1. *What is the stress due to?*

Think dispassionately and try to identify the cause of stress. Is it an illness? Is it an unpleasant job? Is it marital disharmony? Is it a delinquent child? Is it a financial problem? Is it litigation?

2. Does it really matter?

Ask yourself whether you really have a major problem on hand, or is it merely an inconvenience. Viewed from the yogic standpoint, most of our 'problems' cease to matter because:

(a) Our wants are reduced. We realise that fulfilment of no worldly desire is going to bring lasting happiness. Therefore, even the desires that persist lose their intensity.

(b) Our bitterness towards people is gone. When we start viewing everyone as a manifestation of the Divine, we can see some good in all, and overlook what we think is evil in them.

(c) When things don't seem to be going our way, we feel that our way of looking at things may be wrong. The unseen divine hand is there behind all happenings, and therefore whatever happens is always the best that could happen.

(d) Our limited areas of concern become to us a very small part of the much larger design of the Divine. Viewed from that angle, our way of looking at right and wrong, success and failure, victory and defeat, becomes utterly meaningless. In fact, our very existence as an individual ceases to matter. God's work does not depend on us. He will use us as an instrument for carrying on a bit of His work as long as He pleases. But the work will continue on schedule even if we are no more.

Reviewing our own past experience also helps in putting things in the right perspective. Although the emotions associated with past events subside, memory of the events stays with us for ever.

(a) Think of some strong desire you have had in the past. If it was fulfilled, did it bring lasting happiness? If it did not, what makes you think that fulfilment of the present desire will? If the desire of the past was not fulfilled, did it really matter? If it did not, what makes you think that fulfilment of the present desire is terribly important?

(b) Think of some problem about which you were once very worked up. Now when you think back, doesn't it sound quite silly that you got so emotional about it. You might have paid a heavy price for it, say, in terms of your health. Was it worth it? How did the problem finally resolve: was it entirely because of your efforts? Then, why not keep your cool. The present problem will also resolve, and possibly, at least partly, irrespective of your efforts.

> **NOTHING LASTS FOR EVER**
> The good thing about bad things is that they come to an end.
> The bad thing about good things is also that they come to an end.

3. *Can something be done?*

If you think there is nothing that can be done about the problem, do at least one thing: relax! However, generally there is something that can be done. The solutions that suggest themselves fall in one out of two categories.

(a) <u>Changing the circumstances</u>

Having identified the culprits in our circumstances, we feel that if we deal with them appropriately, our problems will be over. Although logical, this approach has very limited value for a variety of reasons. First, our circumstances may be beyond our control. Secondly, culprits in our circumstances may be some persons, and it is almost impossible to make people change. Finally, even if our circumstances change, we will soon discover something new in our new circumstances, which now seems responsible for a new problem!

(b) <u>Changing our attitude to circumstances</u>

We cannot change others but we can change ourselves. We can look at circumstances differently, and that can take all the misery away although the circumstances remain exactly the same. The yogic perspective helps us in doing exactly that. The freedom to look at our circumstances as we choose is the ultimate freedom which nobody can take away from us. Even Hitler could not take that freedom away from the Jews – some of them retained their sanity and sense of humour even in concentration camps. We can *always* refuse to be miserable. There are very few situations in which emotional conflicts cannot be resolved through a proper attitude. It is often believed that attitudes seldom change. Although it is difficult, it is possible to change one's attitude. Many have done it, and so can you.

> **DONT'T WORRY, BE HAPPY**
> Dont't worry about things which you can do nothing about.
> Don't worry about things which you can do something about: just do it

Specific measures for stress relief

Besides the above general outline of stress management, some specific measures may offer additional relief.

1. *Asanas*

Physical activity, by itself has stress-relieving effects. And asanas, specially if done with the right attitude, are more relaxing than other forms of physical activity. Thirdly, some asanas, such as shavasana, are particularly relaxing. Finally, a brief period of intense stretching of the body followed by sudden total relaxation of the body has a marked relaxing effect on the mind as well. This technique, called instant relaxation technique (Nagendra & Nagarathna, 1997), may be practised several times a day, even while sitting on a chair. Alternate nostril breathing is also a relaxing practice which can be carried out anytime, anywhere.

2. *Meditation*

About twenty minutes of meditation, preferably twice a day, but at least once, is very relaxing, and has a carry over effect during the rest of the day.

3. *Stay busy*

Work is an excellent emotional anaesthetic. If you keep yourself busy with work, or hobbies, and get absorbed in them, you will have little time to worry. On the other hand, an idle mind tends to brood over problems, which in turn aggravates stress.

4. *Help someone*

Try to find someone else whom you can help – someone with a worry, someone who is sick, children whom you can teach, or a philanthropic organisation in need of volunteers. Apart from being good in itself, such activities relieve stress in several ways. First, you realise that you are not the only one with problems, and that makes you feel better. Misery loves company, as they say. Secondly, you may find that your problems are very small as compared to other people's problems. A person stops complaining about not having shoes when he finds a person not having feet. Finally, getting involved in someone's problems reduces our absorption with our little self. Self-absorption is a potent means of self-torture.

5. *Express yourself*

Find a way of expressing your feelings. For example, you may start writing a diary. If you are more creative, you may find self-expression in writing poetry or in painting.

6. *Talk to someone*

Talking our problems over with someone makes us feel lighter. We may also get some good advice, but what we need most is someone to listen to us. However, we cannot open ourselves to everyone. The person in whom we confide should have the following qualities:

- (a) He should be your well wisher.
- (b) He should have empathy, or at least sympathy.
- (c) He should be neutral. For example, a girl having marital problems should avoid talking to her parents because they are not neutral.
- (d) He should be a good listener.
- (e) He should have the time to listen, and should be willing to spare the time.

(f) He should be able to keep secrets.

(g) He should be wise enough to give good advice

A person with all the above qualities is not easy to find. If you have one such person in your life, you are indeed lucky. If you do not have even one such person in life, there is nothing to feel bad about: you have plenty of company. If you do not have a friend or relative to confide in, consult a doctor, preferably a psychiatrist, or a counselor. These are good supports, but have limitations. Their relationship with us is professional rather than emotional, and they may charge us for their time. However, there is one support having all the desirable qualities in a confidante plus more: God. He is always available to all of us. We can share all our problems with Him, and receive His guidance in the form of our inner voice. He loves us, and has all the time to listen to us. If we find it difficult to relate to a nameless, formless God, we can relate to His human forms – an avatar, prophet, guru – anyone in whom we have faith, and with whom we have established a bond. The danger here is that we may mistake our own misguided impulses for His voice, and thereby find justification for wrong deeds. To recognise His voice, we need receptivity and complete sincerity – anything which smacks of egoism, selfishness or hatred cannot be His voice. He loves all of us, and therefore His voice is based on unqualified love even for our opponents. Moreover, following only His voice can bring us lasting inner peace and happiness. If we cheat ourselves and mistake our own voice for His will, we get no lasting solution to our miseries.

Cast all your anxiety on Him because He cares for you.
— THE BIBLE

Take refuge in Me alone. I will deliver thee from all sin and evil, do not grieve.
— LORD KRISHNA, TO ARJUNA, IN THE *GITA* (18 : 66)

The best friend one can have – isn't he the Divine, to whom one can say everything, reveal everything.
— THE MOTHER (OF SRI AUROBINDO ASHRAM)

CONCLUSION

The key to stress relief is changing ourselves so that we can view the problem, our circumstances, and the people around us in a new light. Yoga provides us a new way of viewing our situation primarily because of two reasons. First, it sets high goals for us, as a result of which many small things cease to matter. Second, it makes us think positively because we start seeing a divine spark in all persons and the divine hand behind all events.

Frequently Asked Questions

1. *Isn't the yogic approach ideal but not practical?*

   If we can build up the courage to put an ideal into practice, the ideal becomes practical.

2. *Isn't it very difficult to maintain one's cool when one knows others are clearly wrong?*

   Yes, it is difficult. But it is good to remember that after some time you may yourself feel that the other person was not entirely wrong. If you keep that possibility always open, it will be easier to keep your cool.

3. *What can one do when others are unreasonable?*

   Others will behave according to their nature, you should behave according to your nature. The world is made up of many types: that is what makes it an interesting place. Do not react to unreasonable people. As the Mother (of Sri Aurobindo Ashram) has said, '…go on doing what one has to do with simplicity and sincerity.'

4. *If I do whatever others want, won't I be reduced to nothing?*

   You will not only be reduced to nothing, you will become a nervous wreck. The reason is that you cannot please everybody because different people may expect entirely different things from you. The key is to continue doing what is right with simplicity and sincerity without trying to change others. Regarding being nothing – it is good to remember that we *are* nothing: our abilities are a gift from God; our actions are the result of His choosing us as instruments for specific tasks; and our wealth, power, position and prestige are transient mirages – here today, and gone tomorrow.

5. *If I am very good, won't others take undue advantage of me?*

Look around carefully to see who are really the happiest persons around you: aren't they the ones who pour out love indiscriminately to one and all? Living a good and simple life is far easier and happier than being driven by desires, jealousy, hatred and attachment.

6. *If I consider everybody to be a manifestation of God, and all that happens to be the best possible, won't I lose my sense of good and evil?*

First, the people: we shall not hate anybody because everyone is a manifestation of God. But we can retain our disapproval for their evil deeds. We have to learn to differentiate a person from his acts. We should hate what is wrong, but not the wrongdoer.

Second, the events: all what happens is for the best. We can retain our disapproval for evil together with the understanding that even the evil may eventually lead to a good outcome. We have to learn to differentiate an act from its outcome. We should hate what is wrong, but we can still believe that its outcome may be good. The outcome is a part of a large design which is unknown to us and beyond our comprehension. Therefore we are incapable of judging the outcome, just as we cannot judge just one piece in a large and complex puzzle.

7. *If whatever has to happen will happen, why should I do anything?*

   What we do has two aspects: our work, and our efforts to solve a problem.

   We should continue doing our work because it is our good fortune that we have been chosen to make a contribution to God's programme for the world.

   We should also make reasonable efforts to solve our problems in keeping with the guidance provided by God's voice. Only by doing that we can earn His grace.

   However, since we cannot control the outcome of our work or effort, we should remain detached from them so that we can accept even apparent failure cheerfully.

   If the choice is between being attached and being lazy, it is better to work and be attached even if it means suffering emotionally from the outcome.

8. *How can one solve the problem of sleeplessness?*

   Sleeplessness (or insomnia) is a common, prominent and very troublesome symptom of mental stress. Leave all your problems and cares to the God, Goddess, Guru, or anyone in whom you have faith. Visualise the pillow as His/Her lap. Feel the comfort that the child feels in the mother's lap. Stop any thoughts because they are of no use in solving problems. No problem will go away just by brooding over it at night. Regular meditation during the day should improve your capacity to stop thoughts at will. All this should generally ensure sound sleep within a few minutes. However, do not think about it – thinking about sleep will prevent sleep. Finally, don't worry about sleeplessness. The worry will only make it persist. An occasional night passed with insufficient sleep will not have any lasting effect on health. It will be made up by longer sleep the next night, or the night after that. For more details, see Chapter 6.

For Further Reading

1. Richard Carlson, *Don't Sweat the Small Stuff... and It's All Small Stuff: simple ways to keep the little things from taking over your life*. New York: Hyperion, 1997.
2. Norman Cousins, *Anatomy of an Illness as Perceived by the Patient*. New York: WW Norton, 1979.
3. Swami Gokulananda, *How to Overcome Mental Tension*. Calcutta: Ramakrishna Mission Institute of Culture, 1997.
4. H.R. Nagendra & R. Nagarathna, *New Perspectives in Stress Management*. Bangalore: Vivekananda Kendra Yoga Prakashan, 4th edition, 1997.
5. Dean Ornish, *Love and Survival: 8 pathways to intimacy and health*. New York: HarperPerennial (a division of HarperCollins), 1999.
6. Bernie S. Siegel, *Peace, Love and Healing: the path of self-healing*. London: Arrow Books, 1990.
7. *Health and Healing in Yoga. Selections from the Writings and Talks of the Mother*. Pondicherry: Sri Aurobindo Ashram, 1979.

Lifestyle Disorders

...*knowledge, when it goes down to the root of our troubles, has in itself a marvellous healing-power as it were*

SRI AUROBINDO

8

The Mother of Many Maladies

Gluttony is an emotional escape, a sign that something is eating us.

PETER DE VRIES

Being overweight is not merely a cosmetic problem. It is a highly visible signal that the owner of the excess baggage is at high risk of getting a depressing cluster of dreaded diseases. What is disturbing is that the problem is growing at an alarming rate. Surveys done in Indian cities have revealed that about one-third of adults are overweight. Further, in these cities, about one-third of 10-15 year-olds belonging to affluent families are overweight: the proportion is likely to increase by the time these adolescents turn into adults. Urban India is promising to catch up with Europe and North America where half the adults today are overweight.

WHAT MAKES US PUT ON WEIGHT?

Although obesity is a heterogeneous disorder with a variety of root causes, there is one thing common to every person who puts on weight, and that is *energy imbalance*. The energy intake has to exceed energy expenditure for a person to put on weight. The imbalance may be created by excess intake (eating too much), or low expenditure (physical inactivity), or a combination of both.

Food

In the ultimate analysis, what makes us put on weight is energy intake in excess of expenditure. Energy-giving nutrients are carbohydrates, fats and proteins. Therefore, eating too much of just about any food can make us fat. Cows can grow fat by eating too much grass although grass hardly contains any fat but has lots of fibre. But all the same, there are some finer points which make what we eat as important as how much we eat.

Fat

Food with a high fat content is more likely to make us put on weight for a variety of reasons. First, fat is a concentrated source of energy. On a weight-for-weight-basis, fats give about twice as much energy as carbohydrates or proteins. Second, fatty foods taste good, and, therefore, it is tempting. Who has not experienced the irresistible urge to take, 'just one more' pakora or some other fried namkeen, and end up eating far too many 'one mores'? Finally, to convert carbohydrates or proteins into fat, the body at least has to spend some energy. Hardly any energy is needed to store fat as it is.

Sugar

When sugar is added to any food, it makes it more palatable without making any perceptible difference to its volume, while at the same time adding to its energy content. Hence eating a food sweetened with sugar is a double disaster: the food has more calories, and we eat more of it.

Fibre

Dietary fibre is the tough packing material in which nature packs plant cells. The packing gets disrupted by chewing and churning, but does not get digested. Since it does not get digested, it does not give us any energy. Fibre prevents us from putting on weight in many ways. First, fibrous foods are rough and tough, and therefore, take time and effort to chew. To some extent, we eat till we feel we have been eating long enough. Studies suggest that, on an average, we feel we have eaten enough after eating for about twenty minutes, irrespective of how much energy we have ingested. Hence a fibrous food, which takes longer to eat, tends to cut down the amount of food eaten. For example, one burfi, one vada, one samosa and a cup of tea are not difficult to have, and would contain about 500 calories. To get 500 calories from apples, one would need about 800 grams of apples, which is the weight of about seven apples. Very few would find it easy to have seven apples at one sitting (Fig. 8.1). Secondly, fibre adds to the bulk of the food. Further, because of the tendency of fibre to soak water, it swells up to form a viscous mass.[1] Hence, fibre swells up in the stomach and we feel full. If we feel full, we think it is time

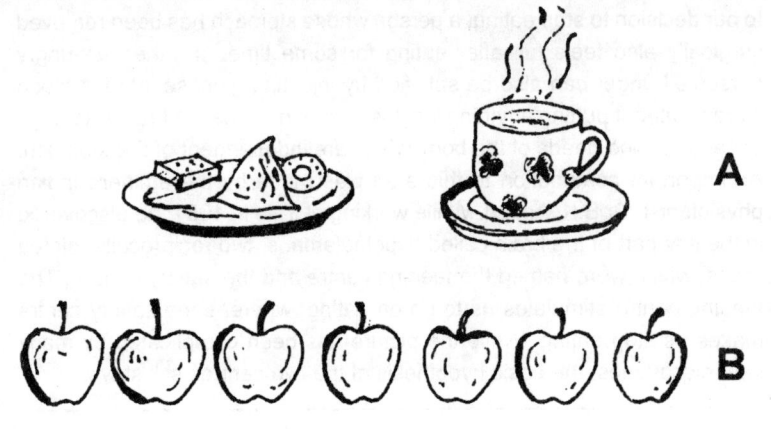

Fig. 8.1. *Foods illustrated in A and B provide the same amount of energy (500 calories each), and yet how different they are.*

---

[1] Soak some ispaghula husk *(isabgol)* or some pectin in water for a few minutes to see how the fibre swells up by holding water and what the consistency of the gel is.

to stop eating. Finally, fibrous foods are not palatable. Sugar, the most refined, fibre-free carbohydrate, is highly palatable. *Maida*, which is almost fibre-free wheat flour, is also quite palatable. In contrast, whole wheat flour is coarse and unpalatable. When juice is extracted from a fruit, the fibre is left behind and is thrown away. That is one reason why the juice is more palatable. The result is that it is easy to drink the juice of four oranges but tiring to eat four oranges. In short, it is very difficult to overeat if our diet consists of fibrous foods.

HOW DO WE KNOW WHEN TO STOP EATING?

Do we stop eating because we feel full, or is it because the brain somehow knows that we have eaten enough? This was a raging controversy about fifty years ago. While it is true that the fullness of the stomach contributes to our decision to stop eating, a person whose stomach has been removed surgically also feels full after eating for some time. Further, a hungry person's hunger can also be satisfied by injecting glucose into his blood stream without putting anything into his stomach. Thus the brain has ways of sensing food needs of the body which are independent of the stomach. An important contribution to this area was made by the eminent Indian physiologist, Dr B.K. Anand. While working at Yale in 1951, he discovered in the tiny part of the brain called hypothalamnus, two reciprocally related areas, which were named the feeding centre and the satiety centre. The feeding centre stimulates us to go on eating, whereas the satiety centre makes us stop eating. While the picture has been complicated by many later discoveries, the basic hypothesis of the two centres still stays.

Exercise

While food is one limb of energy balance, physical activity is another. Like food, physical activity is a necessity for good health. A brisk walk for thirty minutes, or its equivalent, seems to be a reasonable daily 'dose' of exercise.

Psychological factors

If everybody knows eating too much or exercising too little will lead to obesity, why is putting on weight so common? Many factors which may be vaguely grouped under the title 'psychological' enter the picture.

Besides physiological needs, we eat for other reasons. We eat because food offers sensory pleasure. We eat because eating together builds and cements relationships. We eat when we have nothing to do to pass time; and when we have too much to do, food may provide a diversion.

We exercise less because, unlike in case of food, there is no hunger for exercise.[2] On the contrary, physical inactivity is seductively soothing. We seek jobs which involve minimal physical activity. We spend money to buy labour-saving gadgets. And, when we get enlightened, we spend some more money on a treadmill or in the gym so that we can get some exercise. Still we take pride in calling ourselves rational beings!

Stress

Mental stress has effects on eating and physical activity which can work both ways—towards putting on weight, or losing weight. Which way stress will work is too complex to be put into a neat formula. But it is a common experience that one may try to beat stress by overeating. Further, a person under stress may get depressed, and physical inactivity is a prominent feature of depression. Finally, if the stress is due to overwork, there may be little time for exercise. Thus stress can create conditions which promote weight gain. There is also some evidence that stress alters the hormonal status in such a way as to favour deposition of fat, particularly in the abdominal area.

---

[2] This is not strictly true. Those who exercise regularly get addicted to it. Lack of exercise even for a day makes them uneasy, gives them a feeling of having missed something important.

Hormones and genes

Hormones and genes are two convenient scapegoats on which we often depend to avoid feeling guilty for having put on weight. While our constitution might make some of us obese no matter what we do, most cases of obesity are due to 'simpler' reasons as discussed above. When there are indications that deficiency of thyroid hormones, or excess of adrenal cortical hormones may be responsible for obesity, a doctor would order tests to rule out the suspicion and start appropriate treatment.

The role of genes is more complex. Most of the time, it is a large number of genes which together create a tendency towards putting on weight. The tendency is created by having more efficient metabolism so that the person needs less energy. But the central fact remains that there is an imbalance between the energy intake and expenditure.

Another important fact to keep in mind is that obesity running in families does not, by itself, prove that it has a genetic basis. The child eats whatever is available at home. The child tends to copy the food preferences and physical activity choices of the parents. The result is that if the parents are obese, the children also become obese irrespective of genes being involved. As a wag has observed, although fat owners have fat dogs, there is certainly no genetics involved.[3]

DIAGNOSIS OF OBESITY

The most popular criterion for classifying people into 'normal' and 'overweight' is the Body Mass Index (BMI). Mathematically,

---

[3] Hormones and genes have been deliberately underplayed in this book because of two reasons. First, the emphasis here is on things which we can do something about rather than those which we cannot help. Secondly, irrespective of the cause of obesity, every case would benefit from an effort to restore the energy balance. There is no obesity under famine conditions.

$$BMI = \frac{Weight\ (in\ Kg)}{[Height\ (in\ metres)]^2}$$

For example, if a person weighs 60 kg, and his height is 165 cm (1.65 metres), then his BMI = 60/1.65 x 1.65 = 60/2.72 = 22. Using BMI as the criterion, persons having a BMI below 25 are considered normal, those between 25 and 30 are considered overweight but not frankly obese, and those above 30 are considered obese.[4] This is the classification approved by WHO in 1998, and is largely based on western populations. The rationale for the cut-off point of 25 is that above that the risk of diseases associated with obesity increases sharply. But in India, it has been observed that the risk increases sharply above a BMI of 23. The reason is that what increases the risk is the fat content of the body. For the same body weight, Indians have more fat but less muscle than the western populations. Hence an Indian having a BMI of 23 has as much fat as a European or American having a BMI of 25. The higher BMI of the western man is due to his larger muscle mass.[5]

The practical implications of the above discussion are two-fold. First, our short-term policy should be to aim at a BMI between 19 and 23.[6] Second, our long-term policy should be to become a nation that is physically more active. If we are physically active, our muscle mass increases. As our muscle mass increases, our cut-off for a healthy BMI will also start rising. We do not have to do this in order to copy the west. The reason why we should do it is because a larger muscle mass, by itself, also has protective value against the diseases with which obesity is associated.

---

[4] Strictly speaking, the BMI between 18.5 and 24.9 is normal. Persons with a BMI below 18.5 are considered underweight.

[5] These are generalisations based on averages. There are many muscular men (and women) in India, and for them a BMI up to 25 is quite healthy.

[6] At a BMI below 19, the risk for diseases associated with under-nutrition increases sharply.

CONSEQUENCES OF OBESITY

Doctors often predict that a person is likely to get a particular disease in the near future on the basis of blood tests. In these tests they measure substances present in milligram or nanogram concentrations which are known to appear in blood consistently and predictably before the disease manifests itself. Such substances are called markers of the disease. A high concentration of cholesterol is a well-known marker of heart diseases. Obesity is a marker of a huge cluster of diseases, but it does not need a blood test because it is highly visible. It is interesting, however, that we pay greater attention to the reports of blood tests than to a marker staring at us in kilogram quantities. The fact that obesity leads to hypertension, heart disease and diabetes is well known. However, not so well known is the association between obesity and gall bladder stones, menstrual problems and certain cancers. Further, due to mechanical reasons, obesity may also predispose a person to problems associated with the hip and knee joints, and to the obstruction of the air passages during sleep, leading to respiratory distress.

Obesity at an early age

Obesity early in life has particularly sinister implications. First, it has been seen that a child who is born underweight but becomes overweight by the age of five carries an even higher risk of developing the triad of hypertension, heart disease and diabetes than someone who puts on weight later on in life. Secondly, obese children tend to become obese adults. Thirdly, obesity in childhood is also associated with high blood cholesterol levels and poor glucose tolerance (a precursor of diabetes). The result is that obese children are at a high risk of getting hypertension, heart disease and diabetes at a rather young age. The high prevalence of childhood obesity today is one reason why these diseases, traditionally considered midlife or old age problems, are now being seen even in the thirties. Last but not the least, obese children face ridicule and rejection from other children, which may lead to behavioural problems. For a child or teenager, being different from others is a great psychological trauma.

LABORATORY TESTS

Although the diagnosis of obesity itself does not need any laboratory test, doctors ask for some tests in case of obese persons to assess how close he has come to getting some of the diseases associated with obesity. From this point of view it is advisable to get these tests done: fasting blood glucose, blood level of total cholesterol and its fractions, blood level of triglycerides, and an electro-cardiogram. Additional investigations, eg thyroid status, ultrasound of the abdomen, or x-ray of knee joints, may be done if the clinical features of the patient warrant it.

TREATMENT

The treatment of obesity is one area in which whatever is good, is not new; and whatever is new, is not good. The optimum management basically has two well-known, time-honoured components: reduced food intake, and enhanced physical activity. The newer approaches based on drugs and surgery have enough drawbacks to make them the last resorts.

The target weight need not be the ideal weight based on height-weight tables. We are all born different, and some of us will be heavier than the rest while being quite healthy. Therefore, the target should be realistic, based on the person's constitution and hereditary tendency. Weight loss, although short of the ideal, also confers health benefits in terms of an increased sense of well-being and reduced risk for chronic disease.

In overweight growing children, the target should not be weight loss but slower weight gain. For example, an overweight eight-year-old may gain some weight over four years and become a normal twelve-year-old. Severe dietary restrictions in such children to achieve weight loss may interfere with the increase in height. For similar reasons, pregnancy or lactation is not the right time for severe dietary restrictions to achieve weight loss.

Those who are overweight, and also have diabetes, and are taking insulin or tablets for its treatment, should take care that in the process of restricting food they do not let their blood glucose fall to a dangerously low level (hypoglycaemia): for more details, please refer to Chapter 11. Further, losing weight also generally reduces the severity of diabetes with the result that, after weight loss, the dose of insulin or tablets required might be less.

Those who are overweight along with having high blood pressure, may get some relief by merely losing weight. Hence, if they are taking some pills, the dose which they needed earlier might become excessive after losing weight. This fact is important to keep in mind so that the dose can be adjusted promptly lest there should be symptoms of low blood pressure.

Now we shall discuss the two basic strategies for losing weight: dietary restriction and exercise. Of the two, paying attention to the diet is more effective than exercise. Of course, a combination of both is the best treatment.

Diet

For achieving weight loss at a reasonable rate, the daily energy intake should be 500-600 Calories less than the energy expenditure. This is generally achieved through diets which provide 1000-1500 Calories per day. A dietician's help should be sought for converting these figures into a diet which is compatible with the normal eating habits of the person concerned.

In general, however, fats and sugar should be restricted. Fibrous foods should be encouraged: these include whole grains, fruits and vegetables. The intake of fruits and vegetables should be increased: a daily intake of about 500 g of fruits and vegetables is not only acceptable but also desirable. This can be achieved by taking 5-6 helpings of fruits/vegetables per day – one helping at breakfast, two at lunch, one in the evening, and two at dinner. The advantages of liberal fruit and vegetable intake are two-fold. First, they add to the total weight and volume of the diet without adding many calories. Thus they make the diet filling without making it fattening. Secondly, they make the diet balanced by providing vitamins, minerals and dietary fibre. This is an important contribution because other sources of these nutrients are restricted in a reducing diet. Of course, it goes without saying that fruits and vegetables should preferably be had uncooked or boiled. If cooked in fat or fried, vegetables will contain calories.

A few tips which will help one to stick to a diet are given below.

1. Maintain a 'food diary' in which you write down everything you eat. This will make you conscious of the snacks in-between meals which very often ruin sensible diets.
2. The whole family should move towards a healthier diet. What is good for losing weight is also good for maintaining normal weight. A healthy diet for one who is overweight is also healthy for others, except that if weight loss is not required, the quantity should match the requirements.
3. The right place for making choices for a healthy diet is the market rather than the kitchen or the dining table. One eats what is available, and what is available at home depends on what is bought in the market.

Some overweight persons have a misguided attraction for crash diets. They feel it is better to 'suffer' a drastic reduction in diet for a few days and be done with it than to practice perpetual self-denial. But, besides being unsafe, this strategy does not work. After the crash diet and impressive weight loss comes the rebound indulgence, and the person is back to square one.

One should also beware of fad diets which try to make losing weight look very simple. No foods have magical slimming properties. Lop-sided diets such as low-carbohydrate or high-protein diets have also not been able to establish their superiority, or even safety. The simplest diet is one which contains all the normal foods but in smaller quantities, and one which compensates for the smaller quantity by a moderate excess of fruits and vegetables is the safest, and at least as effective as any of the complicated diets containing exotic foods or unusual combinations.

An example of a 1200-calorie diet for an overweight person is given below:

Breakfast

Two sparingly buttered slices of bread, 1 boiled egg, one helping of fruit, tea

Lunch

Two chapattis, one bowl of vegetables (say, potato and a green vegetable), half a bowl of dal, half a bowl of curd, a big helping of salad

Evening

One helping of fruit, tea

Dinner

A small helping of rice, one bowl of vegetables (say, spinach), half a bowl of dal, a big helping of salad

If you recollect what you learnt in Chapter 2, you would see that it is based on the principles given in the following table:

Characteristic of a diet	Consequence
Most of the foods in small quantity	Low energy intake
Restricted amount of fat	Low energy intake
Cereal-pulse mixture	Adequate quantity of good quality protein
Liberal intake of fruits and vegetables	Adequate vitamins, minerals and dietary fibre + Filling diet

There are a few additional features of the proposed diet, which are not essential in a reducing diet, but have been introduced deliberately to expose some popular myths. Its fat content is low, but fat has not been completely excluded: even some butter has been allowed on the slices of bread! It is the total energy content of the diet which is important, not the total exclusion of fat. In fact, some amount of fat keeps the diet palatable and acceptable, and imparts satiety value to the diet. Banana, rice and potatoes have also not been excluded because, in themselves, these are not 'fattening foods'. In fact, there is nothing like a 'fattening' or slimming food. It is the energy intake in relation to the energy expenditure which determines the body weight. If the intake exceeds expenditure, any diet, no matter what it includes or what it excludes, will lead to weight gain.

Exercise

It is relatively easy to cut down on energy intake by 500 Calories by eating less. But to increase energy expenditure by 500 Calories needs a lot of exercise, a lot more than most people find convenient or pleasant. Therefore the quantitative contribution of exercise to tilting the energy balance is relatively small. But that does not mean exercise is not important. Exercise is important and necessary for all – whether thin or fat, young or old, whether wanting to lose weight, or wanting to gain weight. Physical activity promotes health in general, especially cardiovascular fitness (Chapter 5).

There are two ways to increase physical activity: by making a conscious effort to increase its share in one's daily life, and by creating a specific slot for exercise itself. Both are important. One may deliberately choose to make small errands walking instead of using a vehicle for them. One may choose the staircase instead of the lift. And, if the major part of a long journey has been covered by bus, one may walk the remaining distance instead of waiting for another bus. In addition to these healthy choices, it is also desirable to create a slot for exercise. A brisk walk for thirty minutes, or some other exercise equivalent to it is desirable for all. Those wanting to lose weight may increase the duration of the exercise if they like, and if their health permits.

For exercise to become a part of one's daily routine, it should not be very strenuous. Further, if a person has been sedentary for several years, he should start with mild exercises, and build it up gradually over a few weeks. Finally, if a person has any heart disease or some other major health problem, he should consult his specialist before starting on an exercise programme.

The energy consumption during a few activities is given below to help you form a mental picture of how many calories we burn on some everyday activities and popular exercises.

Activity	Energy consumption		Relative energy consumption*
	(Calories/hour)	(Calories/min)	
Sedentary activities			
Lying down peacefully	60	1.0	1.0
Reading silently	66	1.1	1.1
Sitting	66	1.1	1.1
Sleeping	54	0.9	0.9
Very light activities			
Bathing	168	2.8	2.8
Brushing teeth	138	2.3	2.3
Combing	138	2.3	2.3
Cooking	150	2.5	2.5
Desk work	84	1.4	1.4
Dressing/undressing	120	2.0	2.0
Driving a car	120	2.0	2.0
Dusting	168	2.8	2.8
Eating	90	1.5	1.5
Feeding/dressing a child	138	2.3	2.3
Knitting	138	2.3	2.3
Playing a violin	84	1.4	1.4
Reading aloud	90	1.5	1.5
Sewing/stitching/tailoring	90	1.5	1.5

Activity			
Shaving	138	2.3	2.3
Standing still	84	1.4	1.4
Talking	72	1.2	1.2
Typing	102	1.7	1.7
Walking (3 km/h)	120	2.0	2.0
Walking upstairs (1.5 km/h)	120	2.0	2.0
Walking downstairs (3 km/h)	150	2.5	2.5
Watching TV	84	1.4	1.4
Writing	90	1.5	1.5
Yogasanas	84	1.4	1.4

Light activities

Driving a motorcycle	180	3.0	3.0
Ironing	180	3.0	3.0
Lab work	180	3.0	3.0
Sex		3.0	3.0
Walking (5 km/h)	210	3.5	3.5

Moderately heavy activities

Cycling (10 km/h)	300	5.0	5.0
Gardening	240	4.0	4.0
Golf	300	5.0	5.0
Walking (6 km/h)	240	4.0	4.0

Heavy activities

Mountain climbing	480	8.0	8.0
Rowing (6 km/h)	480	8.0	8.0
Rowing (18 km/h)	720	12.0	12.0
Running (10 km/h)	600	10.0	10.0
Running (15 km/h)	900	15.00	15.00
Running (25 km/h)		50.0	50.0
Squash	600	10.0	10.0
Swimming (3 km/h)	540	9.0	9.0
Table Tennis	360	6.0	6.0
Tennis	480	8.0	8.0
Walking (8 km/h)	540	9.0	9.0
Walking upstairs (3 km/h)	420	7.0	7.0

Based on data from multiple sources. Figures rounded off and approximate.

*Energy consumption as a multiple of resting energy consumption.

As you would observe, the first column gives the energy consumption in calories per hour. These figures are for an adult weighing about 60 kg. The second column gives the energy consumption in calories per minute. Since a person weighing 60 kg consumes about 60 Cal/hour when relaxed and lying down but not sleeping, the energy consumption in this state comes to about 1 Cal/minute. Thus, if we express the energy consumption for various activities as a multiple of energy consumed at rest, it comes to the same figure as the energy consumption per minute. That is what has been done in the third column. This is a very useful expression because it gives a unit-free figure, and gives a proportionate idea of how strenuous a given activity is. As is seen in the table, a very large number of everyday activities take only one and a half to two times the energy consumed at rest.

THYROXINE IS NOT FOR THINNING

Thyroxine is the product of the thyroid gland. It is well known that one of the symptoms of deficient thyroid function (hypothyroidism) is obesity. The treatment is to take thyroxine in the form of tablets. While every person with hypothyroidism is overweight, very few overweight persons have hypothyroidism. Thyroxine is the treatment for hypothyroidism, not for obesity. Thyroxine should be taken only after the diagnosis of hypothyroidism has been made by a doctor and confirmed through appropriate laboratory tests. The major effect of thyroxine is to step up energy expenditure. But it is undesirable to use this effect of thyroxine simply for losing weight. Using thyroxine when it is not really required has two serious ill effects. First, it leads to loss of muscle tissue as well as fat. Weight should be lost by losing only fat. Secondly, thyroxine taken by a person with normal thyroid function leads to symptoms of excessive thyroxine (hyperthyroidism) such as tiredness, palpitation, feeling too hot, diarrhoea, etc.

YOGA AND BODY WEIGHT

The popular way to analyse this question is to compare yogasanas (physical postures) with other forms of physical exercise in terms of their efficiency for losing weight. From this angle, yoga is not a good choice because yogasanas, in general, are not very strenuous. Further, in a session of yogasanas, quite some time is spent on relaxation in *shvasana* or *makarasana*. Therefore, if one has only thirty minutes available for exercise, many options such as jogging or badminton would lead to greater energy expenditure than yogasanas. But the significance of yoga resides in several other facts. First, yogasanas are better than many other more strenuous exercises in promoting physical fitness and general well-being. Secondly, yoga is suitable for all age groups, even for the elderly, for whom strenuous exercises may be out of the question. If due to limitations such as painful joints or backaches, a person cannot do certain asanas, there are still many more which he can do. Thirdly, yogasanas can be done at home without any equipment in any simple, loose garment: even a night suit is fine. Finally, yoga incorporates both exercise and dietary changes as a part of physical culture. Physical culture includes all those practices which promote physical health. Physical health is given a lot of importance in yoga because it is considered a sacred duty to look after the body which has been given to us for contributing our bit to the divine plan. With this attitude, food becomes one of the requirements for making the body strong and healthy, not a source of sensory pleasure. Therefore, the choice of foods, and the quantity of food consumed, are guided by the needs of the body, not by the greed for what tastes good. Further this prudent choice is made willingly and cheerfully because a person on the path of yoga has discovered lasting peace and joy which are not dependent on fleeting sensory pleasures. If a person reminds himself of these arguments at the beginning of every meal, he will eat only what is good for him, and only as much as he needs. Moreover, he will do it with a sense of delight, not a sense of deprivation. In short, what is good (*shreyas*) also becomes pleasurable (*preyas*).

CLOSING THOUGHTS

It is easy to lose weight but difficult to sustain it. The reason is that there is a tendency to go back to the old ways once the weight is lost. In fact, after losing weight the energy requirements become less than before because now the body has to maintain a smaller mass. For the same reason, the rate of weight loss is fastest at the beginning of a diet and exercise programme. After some weight has been lost, the gap between the energy intake and the expenditure becomes less even if the same diet and level of exercise are maintained. Thus, during the first month more than 1 kg may be lost every week, but after that one may have to be contented with a loss of just 0.5 kg per week. Besides the diet and exercise, it is also important to pay attention to stresses and anxieties which might be responsible for the tendency to overeat. Here again, yoga comes in handy with its potent prescriptions for lasting mental peace.

WHEN A SOLUTION BECOMES A PROBLEM

Life evolved under conditions of unpredictable and erratic food supply. Under those conditions, storing energy in the body as fat was an ingenious way of making the best use of periods of plenty, and surviving lean periods. One could overeat when food was available, store the excess as fat, and mobilise it when food was scarce. But today a large section of humanity is fortunate to have a regular supply of four or more meals every day, and the meals may be tempting enough to promote overeating. Giving in to the temptation once in a while may not do any harm, but if it becomes a regular habit, the result is obesity and all the maladies associated with it.

Frequently Asked Questions

1. *Is it alright for a sedentary person to maintain normal body weight solely by controlling his food intake?*

   It is better than the sedentary person becoming overweight, but the best would be to exercise regularly and also eat a little more. Exercise has benefits which go far beyond its assistance in maintaining weight.

2. *Of the two components of a weight reduction programme, viz dieting and exercise, which is more important?*

   Both contribute to weight loss, but the contribution of dieting is generally greater. However, exercise is important because:
   a. It does make a contribution, and every bit counts,
   b. There is some evidence that regular exercise may raise the rate of energy expenditure even during the non-exercise part of the day, and
   c. Exercise promotes physical fitness and a sense of well-being.

3. *Does the distribution of energy intake between different meals matter so far as change in body weight is concerned?*

   Yes, there is some evidence that the calories consumed during dinner are more likely to be converted into fat than those taken at other meals. The reason possibly is that not much activity follows dinner. Hence there is something to the adage, 'Breakfast like a king, lunch like a prince, and dinner like a pauper.'

4. *Does the number of meals in a day matter so far as body weight is concerned?*

   Yes, there is some evidence that distributing the food into 4-5 meals is less fattening than taking the same quantity in one or two meals. The reason possibly is that if a lot is consumed at a single sitting, it is likely to get deposited as fat. And once deposited, withdrawal may pose problems. Therefore, it is advisable to have small and frequent meals.

5. *How does a variety of foods at a meal affect body weight?*

   In general, a variety is desirable because it helps in achieving adequate intake of all nutrients. But too great a variety can promote weight gain. The reason is that in the process of taking 'at least a little bit' of every available item on the menu, the total quantity of food may exceed the requirements.

6. *Are there some good drugs available for losing weight?*

   If there were any, they would be widely known because of the heavy demand. A new drug comes every few years, and when it has exhausted its promise, yet another one comes along. The drugs belong to one of the following categories:

a. Drugs which reduce the appetite: none of them is safer or more effective than will power.

b. Drugs which increase energy expenditure: none of them is safer and more effective than exercise.

c. Drugs which inhibit digestion: these are a concession to lack of will power. One may eat more because one cannot help it, but leave part of the food undigested so that it does not contribute to energy intake. Apart from being a sophisticated way of wasting food, it also has unpleasant side effects. The most popular, naturally, are the drugs which hamper fat digestion. The undigested fat remains in the intestines. Some of it is excreted in the faeces, making them greasy. Some of the undigested fat is fermented by bacteria. Fermentation produces gas. Therefore the person gets flatulence, and the stool may become, besides being greasy, also frothy and foul smelling.

7. *Is there a surgical treatment for obesity?*

Yes, not one, but several surgical approaches have been tried. However, each of them has problems, worse than those associated with drugs. Just to enumerate some of the operations that have been done: one involves removing a sheet of fat from the abdomen, or sucking it out from wherever it has accumulated. This may give some temporary relief, but if the basic factors that led to obesity remain, the problem will soon be back. Another approach tries to reduce the capacity of the stomach so that the person feels full faster. Losing the storage capacity of the stomach is not free of problems. Finally, the surgeon may try to reduce the effective length of the small intestine (where the final stages of digestion and absorption are carried out) so that all that is eaten is not digested. This approach creates problems similar to those created by drugs which interfere with digestion plus some more because of stagnation in the idle segment of the intestine. In short, surgery is only the last resort, suitable only for the most severe cases, to be considered only after all other options have failed.

8. *What is abdominal obesity, and why is it considered particularly bad?*

   There are two broad categories of obesity depending on where the fat is predominantly deposited. If the deposit is mainly in the trunk, it is called abdominal obesity: it is more common in men. On the other hand, if the fat is deposited mainly in the buttocks, it is called gluteal obesity, which is common in women. Abdominal obesity is worse because of its extremely close association with diabetes, high blood pressure and heart disease. To prevent abdominal obesity from getting out of hand, one has to watch the waistline. A man whose trousers keep getting tight within a year has something to think about. As a rule of the thumb, the waist of a woman should measure less than 80 cm (31.5 inches), and that of a man less than 90 cm (35.5 inches).

9. *What is leptin?*

   Leptin is one of the natural substances for regulating food intake. It is produced in fat cells, circulates and reaches the part of the brain which regulates food intake (hypothalamus), and triggers mechanisms which reduce food intake. Thus, the greater the accumulated fat, greater the amount of leptin produced and stronger is the inhibition of food intake. In this way, there is a natural check on body weight. It is tempting to use leptin as a drug for losing weight. It has been done but not with much success. The reason is that most obese persons *do not* have a deficiency of leptin. Rather, it seems they have a defect in the hypothalamus which does not let leptin act. In other words, obese persons are leptin-resistant rather than leptin-deficient. The resistance makes leptin given as a drug, just as ineffective as the leptin produced by the person's own fat cells. We do not as yet have a molecular tool for correcting leptin resistance, but today such a tool is not unthinkable.

9

The Silent Killer

It is one thing to prescribe an anti-hypertensive medication for high blood pressure. It is quite another to expand the patient's context of life so that he stops being angry and repressive.

DAVID HAWKINS, MD, PHD

Hypertension, more commonly known as high blood pressure, is the most predictable, persistent and potentially lethal consequence of the unhealthy lifestyle characteristic of the modern civilisation. Blood pressure rises temporarily during exercise as well as anger, but it takes a lot more for high blood pressure to remain high all the time.

WHAT IS BLOOD PRESSURE?

Blood circulates in the body in a network of tubes called blood vessels. The motive force for the movement of blood through the blood vessels is generated by the heart. As the blood moves through the blood vessels, it exerts some pressure on the vessel walls: this pressure is called blood pressure. However, the pressure exerted on the walls of all the blood vessels is not the same. Imagine a device pumping a fluid into a network of tubes (Fig. 9.1). It is easy

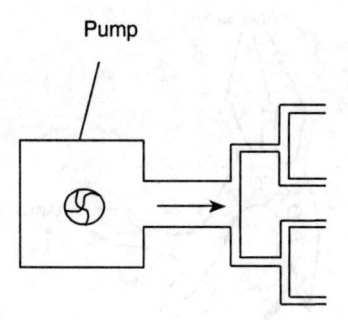

Fig. 9.1. *A diagrammatic representation of a fluid being pumped into a network of tubes.*

to visualise that the fluid pressure will be the highest in the tubes nearest to the pump. In the distant tubes, part of the pressure has already been spent, and hence the pressure is reduced. The heart has four chambers: two atria (singular, atrium) and two ventricles. The chamber that pumps blood throughout the body is the left ventricle (Fig. 9.2). The output of the left ventricle is pumped into a huge blood vessel, curved like a horse-shoe, called the aorta. Just as the stem of a tree gives rise to several branches, the aorta gives rise to a network of branches. The branches enter various organs of the body to supply blood to those organs. The aorta, as well as its initial branches, are called arteries. The pressure exerted on the inside of the arterial walls is called arterial blood pressure, and ordinarily when we talk of blood pressure, it refers to the arterial blood pressure. In hypertension, it is the arterial blood pressure that is above normal.

The arterial blood pressure shows moment-to-moment cyclic fluctuation. This is because the heart is an intermittent rhythmic pump. Suppose the heart rate (or pulse rate) is seventy-five times per minute. It means that the heart is beating once in every 0.8 seconds. Out of 0.8 seconds, the ventricle spends about 0.3 seconds on pumping blood, and about 0.5 seconds on getting filled up with blood (which it can pump during the next 0.3 seconds, and

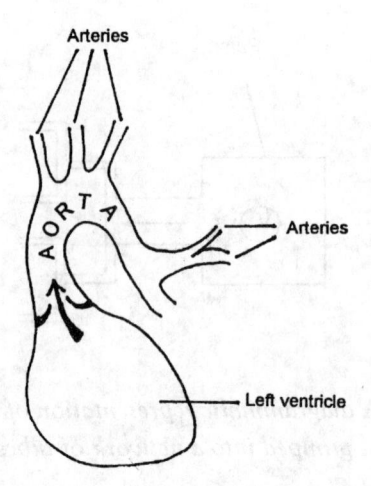

Fig. 9.2. *A schematic diagram of the left ventricle of the heart and the blood vessels into which it pumps blood. The blood pressure is generally measured in the artery which supplies blood to the arm.*

so on). Imagine a pump forcing a fluid into a network of tubes intermittently like the heart (Fig. 9.3). The pressure in the tubes would rise to a peak while the fluid is being pumped. And, when the fluid is not being pumped, the pressure would start falling, and will keep falling till the next pumping motion forces more fluid into the tubes. Thus the pressure in the tubes will have a cyclic fluctuation, but the pressure will always be somewhere between the two extremes: the peak and the bottom. When the doctor takes your blood pressure, he gives you two values, eg 120/80 mm Hg: in this case, 120 is the peak pressure and 80 is the lowest pressure.[1]

---

[1] 'mm Hg' stands for millimetres of mercury. It is the unit in which blood pressure is commonly measured. The peak pressure is technically called the systolic pressure. Systole means contraction; hence systolic pressure is the pressure recorded during ventricular contraction. The lowest pressure is called diastolic pressure. Diastole means relaxation, hence diastolic pressure is the pressure recorded during ventricular relaxation.

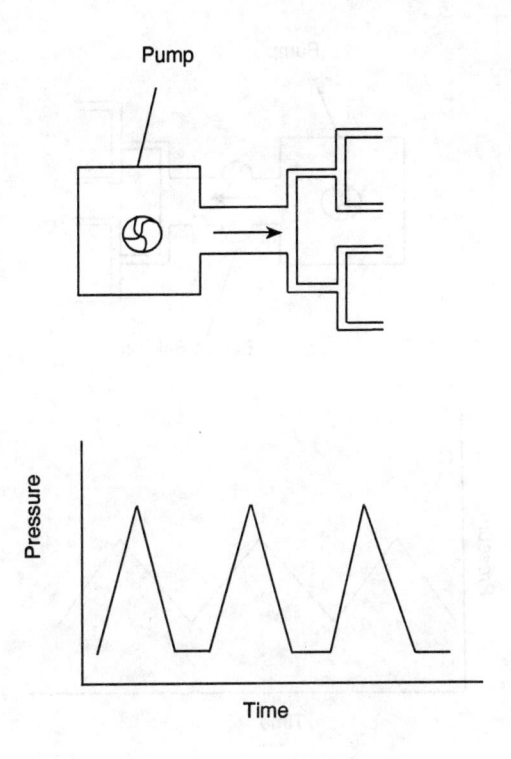

Fig. 9.3. *If fluid is pumped intermittently into a network of rigid tubes, the fluid pressure in the tubes fluctuates synchronously with the pumping action.*

You may feel that the difference between 120 and 80 is rather small in view of the fact that blood is being pumped into the vessels not even half the time (only 0.3 seconds out of 0.8 seconds). In other words, why does the pressure not fall to zero, or at least near zero during ventricular relaxation? The reason is that arteries are elastic tubes. In order to understand the impact of elasticity, imagine a fluid being pumped intermittently into rigid tubes (Fig. 9.3), and the resultant pressure fluctuation in the tubes. Now let us insert an elastic balloon between the pump and the tubes (Fig. 9.4). This has two consequences. First, every time

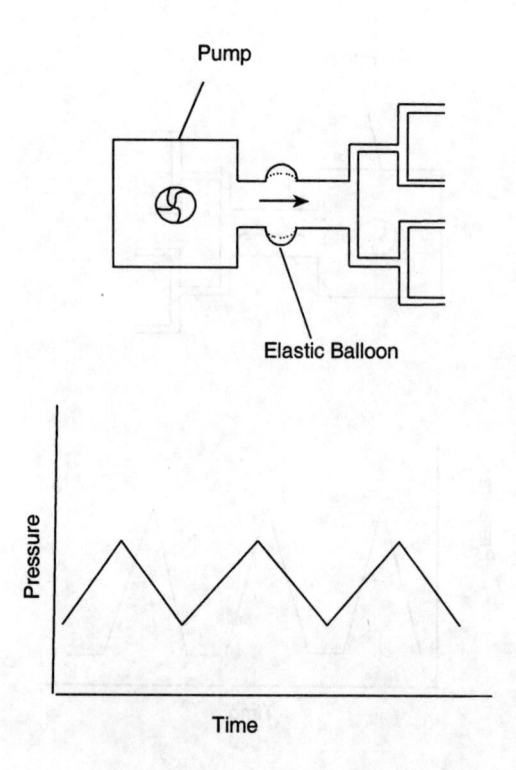

Fig. 9.4. *Everything else being the same as in Fig. 9.3, if an elastic balloon is inserted between the pump and the network of tubes, the pressure fluctuations are markedly reduced.*

the fluid is pumped, not only the fluid runs through the tubes, some of the fluid simply expands the balloon. Hence, the fluid running through the tubes during pumping is reduced. Therefore, the peak pressure is not as high as in Fig. 9.3. Second, when the fluid is not being pumped, the balloon starts shrinking. As the balloon starts closing in on the fluid, the fluid escapes from the balloon and runs through the tubes. Therefore, the fluid keeps running through the tube and continues to exert some pressure on the inside of the tubes even when no fresh fluid is pumped. As a result, the bottom pressure in the tubes is not as low as in Fig. 9.3. In short, the impact of elasticity in the tubes is that the peak pressure is lowered, and the bottom pressure is raised. Thus the difference between the peak and the bottom pressures is reduced. By the same token, if the elasticity of the aorta and large arteries is reduced, the peak pressure is raised, and the gap between the peak pressure and bottom pressure may widen.

What raises the blood pressure?

We saw above that reduction in the elasticity of the aorta and large arteries raises the peak blood pressure. Reduction in the elasticity of the arteries is a normal feature of aging. Besides reduced elasticity, another important factor which raises the blood pressure is narrowing of the arteries. This factor is most effective in raising the bottom pressure, specially when it affects the medium-sized tubes in the arterial tree, which are a little further removed from the pump. Again, it is easy to visualise how it happens. If water is barely dripping out of a gardening hose, it can be made to gush out under high pressure by squeezing the hose or fixing a nozzle at the tip. In the body, narrowing of the arterial tree may result in at least two ways. First, it may result from contraction of the muscles lining the arteries. Secondly, it may result from the deposition of fatty substances in the walls of the arteries. Formation of fatty deposits is a slow and progressive process. But muscle contraction (sometimes called spasm) is relatively quick. If spasm is superimposed on the deposits, it means double trouble. Finally, the blood pressure may rise not due to changes in blood vessels but as a result of an increase in the volume of blood in the blood vessels.

We have so far tried to understand blood pressure by looking at it as the product of blood being pumped into a network of elastic tubes, the diameter of which may vary through a variety of mechanisms. What makes the regulation of blood pressure far more complex in the body is that the pump as well as blood vessels are in touch with the rest of the body and respond to variations in blood flow requirements in different parts of the body. Further, the brain and a variety of hormones change the activity of the pump, the diameter of blood vessels, or the volume of blood circulating in the body, and any of these three affects the blood pressure. As you might have guessed, the involvement of the brain means that thoughts and feelings can also affect blood pressure. Normally this is a good thing, because it ensures that the blood flow through muscles starts increasing while we are planning to go for a walk. Thus the muscles are brought to a state of readiness even before we have left home. But the same arrangement also leads to an unwanted rise in the blood pressure when we are cursing the boss or yelling at our teenaged son.

Before we leave this section, a few words about the importance of the role of the kidneys in the regulation of blood pressure. First, the kidneys regulate the volume of blood circulating in the body by regulating the volume of water and salts excreted in the urine. Second, the kidneys produce a hormone that affects the diameter of blood vessels, the amount of water and salts lost in the urine, as well as how thirsty we feel. Finally, the blood vessels of the kidneys are also affected by the generalised process of deposition of fatty substances in arteries. When that happens, not only does the blood pressure rise due to the narrowing of the blood vessels, the function of kidneys also suffers, which raises the blood pressure further. Hence any kidney-related disease may raise the blood pressure; and high blood pressure may itself lead to a kidney-related disease, which in turn may aggravate the hypertension.

How high is really high?

A person is considered to have hypertension if his blood pressure is above normal. But we have seen that normal blood pressure is not a fixed entity. It rises temporarily during anger and exercise. It may also rise because of the anxiety generated by the doctor recording the blood pressure: this is sometimes called white coat hypertension! Therefore, a person is not labelled hypertensive on the basis of a single high reading. If the reading continues to be high even when the person is relaxed, and feels at home with the doctor and the recording instrument, only then is the person considered hypertensive. For practical purposes, blood pressure less than 120/80 mm Hg is considered optimal, and less than 130/85 mm Hg is also passed off as normal. Blood pressure in the range of 130-139/85-89 mm Hg calls for precautions and frequent check-ups, but is usually not treated. A persistent elevation of blood pressure above 140/90 mm Hg is considered hypertension and needs treatment.

It was once considered that diastolic blood pressure (DBP) higher than 90 mm Hg is more important for diagnosis, and that one need not worry much about a high systolic blood pressure (SBP). This attitude was based on the fact that SBP is more likely to rise temporarily in response to stress or anxiety. But now it has been found that the persistent elevation of SBP also has serious implications, and that SBP may be high even when the DBP is borderline. Therefore, isolated systolic hypertension is also now considered a disease entity which needs medical attention.

If a person is regularly found to have mild or moderate hypertension during some visits, but has normal blood pressure during other visits, he is considered to have labile hypertension. Labile hypertension is a warning that persistent hypertension is likely to follow soon unless adequate precautions are observed.

SYMPTOMS OF HYPERTENSION

By itself, hypertension is generally symptomless. But because of its lethal implications, it is called a silent killer. However, if the blood pressure is very high, it may give rise to headaches. The headache due to hypertension is usually at the back of the head, is at its worst on waking up in the morning and becomes less and less as the day progresses. Long-standing persistent hypertension may cause shortness of breath on exertion, and swelling around the ankles. These symptoms indicate that hypertension has started affecting the heart. Severe hypertension may also be sometimes responsible for dizziness, palpitation, tendency to get tired quickly and sexual inadequacy.

The effect of high blood pressure on blood vessels in different parts of the body may sometimes lead to a variety of manifestations. For example, its effect on the blood vessels of the nose may lead to bleeding from the nose; the effect on the blood vessels of the urinary tract may lead to blood in the urine; and the effect on the blood vessels of the brain may give rise to brief absence attacks. But all these are rather unusual and late manifestations; the most important fact to remember is that high blood pressure begins slowly, silently, without a warning, and progresses stealthily to become a major threat to life and well-being. Therefore, a regular check-up is essential for all adults so that if high blood pressure develops, it can be detected well in time. It is recommended that after the age of thirty, the check-up should be every alternate year, and after the age of forty, every year.

Complications

Although high blood pressure, by itself, is silent, over time it invariably leads to complications which involve some vital organs.

Heart disease

In hypertension, the left ventricle has to pump blood against a higher pressure, and therefore, it has to work harder than normal. This may lead to enlargement of the left ventricle. Secondly, pumping blood against a higher pressure increases the oxygen needs of the heart. This may create a mismatch between the supply and demand of oxygen in the heart. The mismatch may lead to pain in the chest (angina). This aspect will be discussed in detail in the next chapter.

Stroke

A stroke is a general term for the sudden development of a deficit in the function of the brain. It is most often due to an 'accident' (such as rupture or occlusion) involving blood vessels of the brain, and usually manifests as a sudden paralysis, or loss of speech, or loss of vision in selected sectors of the visual field. *Hypertension is the single most important risk factor for a stroke.* Therefore, almost all cases of stroke can be prevented by either preventing hypertension, or by at least treating hypertension promptly.

Retinopathy

The retina is essentially an outpost of the brain. Therefore, the retinal blood vessels are also affected by hypertension. Retinal involvement may eventually lead to blindness, which is also preventable by early detection and treatment of hypertension.

Kidney failure

The intimate relationship between blood pressure and the kidneys has already been referred to. A significant number of persons having high blood pressure end up with kidney disease and may die due to kidney failure.

LABORATORY TESTS IN HYPERTENSION

After the diagnosis of hypertension, it is desirable to do a few laboratory tests in order to know where the patient stands in relation to the major organs which can get affected adversely by the disease. The reports of these initial tests, even if completely normal, should be kept carefully for comparison later on with the reports of tests done during the follow-up. As a follow-up, the following tests should be done once a year:
1. Electrocardiogram (ECG), to check the status of the heart.
2. Fasting blood lipid profile (Blood cholesterol and its fractions, and Blood triglycerides), because of its relevance to heart disease, strokes and diabetes.
3. Fasting blood glucose, because of the frequent association of hypertension with diabetes.

4. Urea, sodium, potassium, chloride and creatinine levels in the blood, to get an idea of the status of the kidneys.
5. Urine examination for presence of protein and red blood cells, also to get an idea of the status of the kidneys.

TREATMENT

Suppose your car breaks down during a journey. If you cannot correct the fault yourself, one way to solve the problem is to hire a few boys to push the car up to a workshop. If the boys get tired before you find a workshop, you can hire another set of boys to continue pushing the car. This is a solution which will work irrespective of the nature of the defect: a blown fuse, a problem with the clutch, or worn-out spark plugs. But it is a temporary solution. A relatively permanent solution will be available in the workshop where the specific defect responsible for the breakdown will be corrected. The various treatments for hypertension also fall in two analogous categories: drugs and lifestyle modification.

Drugs are like the boys hired to push the car. They act on the end result of the problem, and provide a sure but temporary solution. In case of the car, the end result is that the car is not moving. The boys make it move by pushing it. In case of hypertension, the end result is that the blood vessels are narrow; in addition, there is also generally too much of blood to be moved around. Some drugs widen the blood vessels by relaxing their musculature, while other drugs reduce fluid volume by making the kidneys lose additional water in the urine. But the duration of one dose of a drug is limited, say twelve hours. After twelve hours, we have to hire another boy, i.e. take the next dose. So long as we keep taking the pills regularly every twelve hours, the blood pressure will stay normal.

The second mode of treatment, lifestyle modification, is like visiting the workshop. The usual lifestyle factors which lead to high blood pressure are: eating too much of the wrong type of food, too little physical activity, smoking, and prolonged mental stress. Fortunately, just as these unhealthy habits can gradually lead to hypertension, in the same way, correcting them can *gradually* correct hypertension. We have talked about these lifestyle factors in several contexts earlier, especially in relation to obesity. In fact, obesity and hypertension are very closely related. Hypertension frequently follows weight gain. On the other hand, in one who is overweight and hypertensive, simply losing weight brings down the blood pressure.

The analogy of pushing the car versus going to the workshop should not be carried too far though. Lifestyle modification takes time to produce its results. Damage done over decades cannot be corrected in a day. Moreover, if the damage has gone beyond a point, it may be impossible to undo it completely. Therefore, drugs are initially necessary for the treatment of hypertension. Even after lifestyle modification has started having its effect, it may be possible only to reduce the dose of the drugs rather than stop them altogether. That is also a great help because at a low dose the side effects of drugs can be minimised. Drugs may be required for hypertension even if the patient has no symptoms because, as we have seen, damage to several organs may progress silently if no attention is paid to the high blood pressure.

Regarding the exact drugs to be used, it is best to leave that decision to the doctor. He considers several factors, especially the presence or absence of other concomitant diseases, before deciding on the drug to be used for a particular patient. However, if uncomfortable side effects are experienced, the doctor should be informed. He may be able to solve the problem by changing the drug, or by giving a combination of two drugs in low doses, because low doses of two drugs often gives fewer side effects than a single drug in high dose. Fortunately, doctors today have a wide variety of drugs to choose from, and can treat most patients without giving them drugs with uncomfortable side effects.

However, while on drugs, it is important to remember the analogy of pushing the car: a visit to the workshop is important, and should not be neglected. Lifestyle modification is difficult to begin, but once you have experienced the joy it brings, it is so easy to maintain it. How exactly to do it, and what to do, has been discussed already at several places. Fortunately, the lifestyle which is good for maintaining normal body weight is also good for preventing or treating high blood pressure, heart disease, diabetes, and a variety of other problems.

Frequently Asked Questions

1. *Is it normal for the blood pressure to rise with age?*

    Yes, and no. Yes, because if we take the blood pressure of thousands of apparently healthy persons belonging to various age groups, the blood pressure of older individuals is higher. But most such studies have been done within the last one hundred years in the western world which has had a rather unhealthy lifestyle during this very period. The few studies that have been done on the populations which have remained insulated from the impact of modern civilisation have shown that the blood pressure does not have to rise with age. The single most important factor in the lifestyle that leads to age-related rise in blood pressure is dietary salt. Some experts go to the extent of saying that if you add no table salt at all to your food, your blood pressure at age seventy will be exactly the same as it was at seventeen.

2. *Is hypertension a hereditary disease?*

    Like obesity, hypertension also runs in families. What is inherited, however, is not a gene which will definitely produce hypertension, but rather a set of genes which produce a tendency towards developing hypertension. The expression of the tendency depends on the lifestyle. If there is an inherited tendency towards hypertension, and the lifestyle is unhealthy, severe hypertension is sure to develop rather early in life. On the other hand, a healthy lifestyle can delay and blunt the expression of the inherited tendency. In any case, heredity is something which is not in our hands. It is better to do what we can, and not to worry about things which we can do nothing about. Worry will only increase the chances of hypertension! An inherent tendency towards hypertension from birth is not necessarily due to genetic factors. A full-term baby born underweight also has a tendency towards high blood pressure, heart disease and diabetes. The tendency has maximum chance of expressing itself if the child grows overweight by the age of five. Underweight children are generally born to malnourished mothers. Therefore, it is important to look after women's nutrition, not only for their own sake but also for that of the next generation. Low body weight at birth and overweight in childhood is a very dangerous combination.

3. *Should a person having hypertension stop having salt?*

Hypertension is of two types: salt-sensitive and salt-insensitive. The type of hypertension a person has can be best determined by giving the salt-free diet a trial for about four weeks. If the blood pressure comes down, the diet may be continued. Otherwise, the person can continue taking the normal quantity of salt unless the doctor has advised salt-restriction due to some other reason. Since about sixty per cent of persons having hypertension respond favourably to salt-restriction, in practice, salt-restriction (not complete salt omission) is more or less standard advice in hypertension.

4. *What are the special implications of hypertension during pregnancy?*

This question has two aspects. First, if a woman having hypertension gets pregnant, she needs frequent monitoring because of the additional risk of complications. Further, if she is on medication for hypertension, a change may be required because some of the drugs used for high blood pressure are not safe for the foetus.

Secondly, among the women whose blood pressure is normal before pregnancy, a few develop high blood pressure during pregnancy. The treatment depends on the severity of the hypertension, and whether it is accompanied by the presence of protein in the urine (which indicates involvement of the kidneys). With current advances in treatment, the pregnancy can continue in most of these cases, and the safety of both the mother and the foetus can be achieved. However, all such cases need close monitoring and appropriate treatment, and may also need an expert to decide when to terminate the pregnancy or induce delivery. All cases of pregnancy-induced hypertension regain normal blood pressure soon after delivery.

5. *Can oral contraceptive agents (birth control pills) induce hypertension?*

Yes, they can, but it is much less of a problem now with newer pills having a smaller dose of oestrogen. Pills produce hypertension mainly in those susceptible to it for reasons like their age, obesity, family history, etc. The blood pressure returns to normal within six months of stopping the pills. A woman who gets pill-induced hypertension should take it as a warning that she is susceptible to the problem. Therefore, she should not only stop the pill, but also start appropriate lifestyle modification immediately as a preventive measure.

6. *What is low blood pressure?*

Having dangerously low blood pressure all the time the way hypertensives have high blood pressure is almost unknown. What is pretty common, however, is to have short attacks of low blood pressure. The characteristic feature of the attack is fainting, which in turn is due to reduced blood flow to the brain.

About half the attacks of fainting are due to, what is technically called a vasovagal attack. The attack may be precipitated by standing still for a long time, an emotional or stressful situation (eg seeing blood), hunger, severe pain, hot environment, or alcohol. Generally there is an initial warning in the form of light-headedness, dizziness, sweating, a feeling as if the floor or surrounding objects are swaying, or a black out. The warnings may last a few seconds to a minute or so. The right thing to do is to pay attention to the warning, and just lie down (or at least sit down) wherever you are. That makes it possible for the heart to pump blood to the brain without having to work against gravity. The result is generally a quick recovery. Of course, the person should keep lying down for some time to prevent a second attack. If the attack has been precipitated by heat, the person is likely to have sweated quite a lot, and should be given lemonade with salt (*nimboo-pani*). If no attention is paid to the warnings, the person loses consciousness and falls: this is nature's way of forcing the person to lie down, but it can result in expensive treatment because the person may get badly injured while falling.

Hypotension (or low blood pressure) may also be precipitated by change of posture. If a person who has been lying down stands up suddenly, the heart has to adapt to the additional load imposed by gravity. If it cannot do so rapidly, blood pressure may fall leading to a few brief warnings followed by loss of consciousness as discussed above. This happens commonly in the elderly, or in patients taking drugs for high blood pressure. The treatment is simple and consists of a precaution which every person above the age of fifty should take because postural hypotension can happen to anybody. And, the first time it happens, it could take a person unawares and lead to a fall. The precaution to be taken is to cultivate the habit of getting up slowly, systematically and carefully. Take your time while changing the posture from horizontal to vertical. Change the posture in two distinct steps: lying to sitting, and sitting to standing, with a short gap between the two steps. Finally, take care to get the support of a wall, a piece of furniture, or a door handle while changing the posture from sitting to standing.

Finally, hypotension may be triggered in some men by a tight collar, especially while turning the head. This happens because the tight collar presses on a sensitive structure in the neck, which in turn leads to hypotension as a reflex. The treatment is obvious: wear a loose collar.

7. *Does yoga help cure hypotension?*

Yes, it does, because yogic postures exercise cardiovascular reflexes. By sharpening the reflexes, the risk of hypotension can be minimised in most situations. However, yoga only slows the process of aging: it does not stop it altogether. Therefore, the precaution of changing the posture correctly is still worthwhile. Doing simple things like the change of posture with full consciousness is also a part of yoga!

10

The Heart of the Matter

'Healing' is when we use our pain or illness as a catalyst to begin transforming our lives – healing our inner pain and our relationships, our hearts and our souls.

DEAN ORNISH, MD

History shows that as nations progress towards industrialisation and economic well-being, communicable diseases decline and life expectancy increases, but morbidity and mortality due to non-communicable diseases increase in relative as well as absolute terms. Coronary artery disease, commonly known as heart disease, is a major non-communicable disease belonging to this category. The improvement in life expectancy and the changing disease pattern in India during the last few decades indicate that history seems to be repeating itself here. Coronary artery disease is a major public health issue in India today, and the problem will grow unless we adopt a healthier lifestyle.

CORONARY ARTERIES

The heart pumps blood into the aorta. The aorta divides itself repeatedly like the stem of a tree into branches called arteries.

Arteries are distributed all over the body (Fig. 10.1). An artery going to a part of the body carries blood to it. Blood supplies nutrients and oxygen, and takes away carbon dioxide and other waste products (Fig. 10.2). If the blood supply to an organ is blocked, it does not get nutrients and oxygen, and waste products accumulate. Under these conditions, the organ soon dies. You may think that the heart need not have arteries because it is itself full of blood. But that is not true because blood in the chambers of the heart cannot meet the needs of the entire thickness of the heart. Dr Deepak Chopra has coined an analogy to explain this point: a bank employee handles a lot of money, but still needs a salary to look after his own requirements. The requirements of the heart are met by a set of arteries called coronary arteries (Fig. 10.3). Thus coronary arteries are arteries which supply blood to the heart.

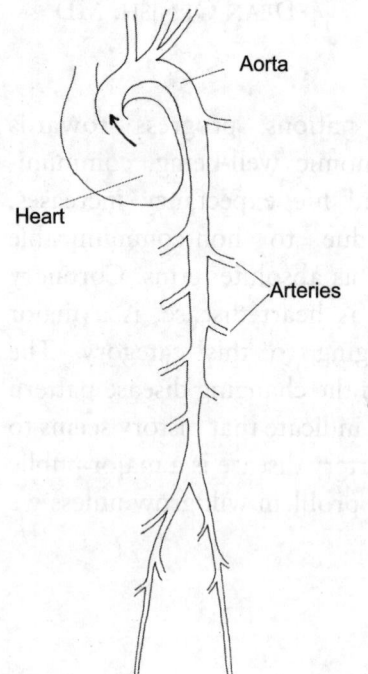

Fig. 10.1. *The heart pumps oxygen-rich blood into the aorta. The aorta divides into branches (arteries) which are distributed all over the body.*

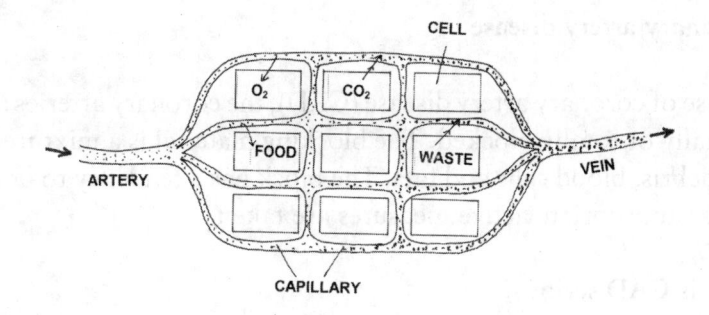

Fig. 10.2. *After an artery enters an organ, it eventually divides into a web of capillaries. Capillaries come very close to cells constituting the organ. Oxygen and nutrients diffuse out of the capillary blood to enter the cells. Carbon dioxide and other waste products diffuse out of the cells to enter capillaries. Blood leaves the organ in a vein.*

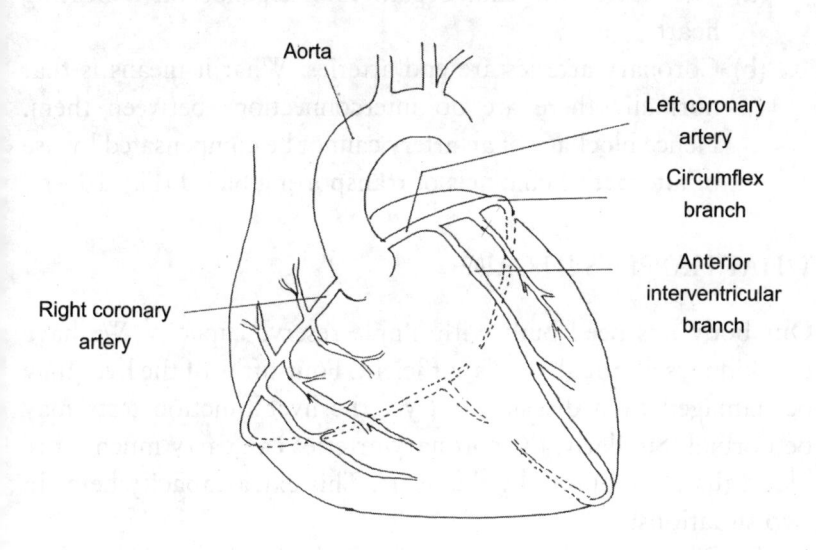

Fig. 10.3. *The coronary arteries supply blood to the heart. As shown here, they are the first pair of arteries arising from the aorta. The three arteries most commonly blocked in CAD are (a) right coronary artery, (b) circumflex branch of left coronary artery, and (c) anterior interventricular branch of left coronary artery.*

Coronary artery disease

In case of coronary artery disease (CAD), the coronary arteries are partially or totally blocked. The blocking material is a mixture of cell debris, blood cells and fats. The block has a tendency to grow unless appropriate active measures are taken.

Why is CAD serious?

The blockage of coronary arteries in CAD is due to a process called atherosclerosis. Atherosclerosis is a generalised process which affects arteries in several organs. But the blockage of arteries due to atherosclerosis is not equally serious in all parts of the body. Blockage of coronary arteries is serious because:
  (a) The heart is a vital organ. Life depends on a beating heart.
  (b) Coronary arteries are end arteries. What it means is that normally there are no interconnections between them. Hence blockage of an artery cannot be compensated by use of alternative channels of transporting blood (Fig. 10.4).

WHAT HAPPENS IN CAD?

Our body has been built with ample reserve capacity. We have two kidneys although one is sufficient. Four-fifths of the liver may be damaged by a disease, and yet the liver function tests may be normal. Similarly, the coronary arteries can carry much more blood than is required by the heart. This extra capacity helps in two situations:
  (a) While exercising, the heart works harder, and therefore needs more blood.
  (b) In CAD, blockages in coronary arteries may remain unnoticed even when the cross-sectional area of coronary arteries is only half of normal.
It follows that the adequacy of coronary blood flow is

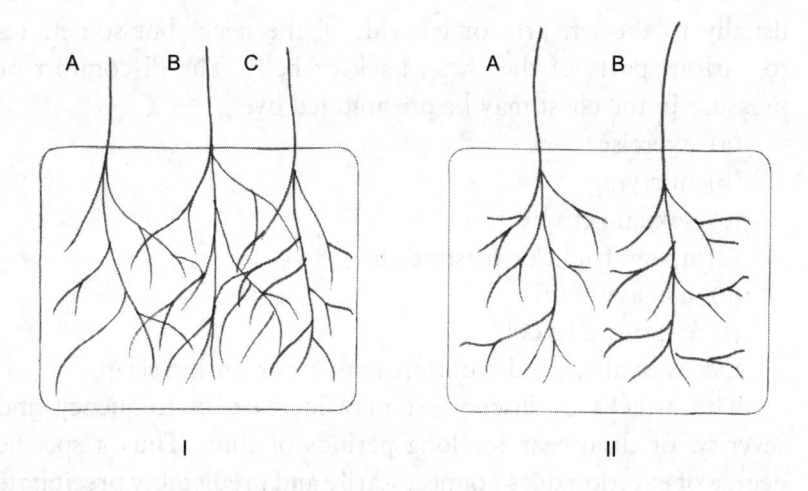

Fig. 10.4. *A diagrammatic comparison of two types of organs, I and II.*
In organ I, there are three arteries, A, B and C. If the blood flow through artery B is blocked, the organ does not suffer because arteries A and C have an overlapping area of distribution and also some cross connections with branches of B.
In organ II, arteries A and B have independent areas of distribution. Therefore blocking of an artery leads to damage of the area dependent on it for blood supply. Arteries A and B are called end arteries.
The situation in the heart is similar to that shown in II.

relative. It is essentially a question of the balance between supply and demand. So long as the blood supply is able to meet the demand, all is well. When the supply is insufficient for the needs, the heart complains. The heart lodges its complaint through pain in the chest. Thus partly blocked coronary arteries may be able to supply enough blood when the person is at rest but not during physical exercise. Therefore the commonest complaint in CAD is chest pain during exercise.

The pain in the chest of CAD is most often felt as heaviness or pressure rather than pain. It increases to a peak and then comes down, a typical cycle occupying one to five minutes. It radiates

usually to the left arm or left side of the neck, but sometimes to various parts of the chest, back or belly. The discomfort or pressure in the chest may be precipitated by:
  (a) exercise
  (b) hurrying
  (c) sexual activity
  (d) anger, fright or frustration
  (e) a heavy meal
  (f) exposure to cold
Occasionally, the discomfort may occur during sleep.

The attacks of discomfort may increase in frequency and severity, or disappear for long periods of time. Thus a specific degree of exertion does not necessarily and predictably precipitate the attack.

> A feeling of intense pressure or tightness in the chest which is precipitated by exertion and relieved by rest may signal CAD.

LABORATORY TESTS IN CAD

The commonly performed tests for determining the severity and characteristics of the disease in a patient having CAD are briefly described below.

Blood cholesterol

High blood cholesterol is a major risk factor for CAD. Measures which reduce blood cholesterol also reduce the risk of getting CAD. Therefore blood cholesterol is used both for determining the degree of risk in an individual and for evaluating the effect of treatment. High levels of the LDL fraction and low levels of the HDL fraction of blood cholesterol predict CAD even better than total blood cholesterol. The interpretation of blood cholesterol is given in Table 1.

TABLE 1. INTERPRETING BLOOD CHOLESTEROL

	Total blood cholesterol	LDL cholesterol	HDL cholesterol
Desirable	< 200 mg/dL	< 130 mg/dL	> 60 mg/dL
Borderline	200-239 mg/dL	130-159 mg/dL	36-60 mg/dL
Undesirable	> 240 mg/dL	> 160 mg/dL	< 35 mg/dL

Based on the second NCEP report (1994).

Electrocardiogram (ECG)

If a part of the heart has been permanently damaged due to lack of blood flow, it gives rise to changes in the ECG (Fig. 10.5). Additionally, transient changes are also seen during the periods when blood flow is less than the demand. The transient changes may be detected if an ECG is done during angina, or may be precipitated during a `stress test' (see below).

Stress tests

These tests are based on the principle that till the narrowing (stenosis) of coronary arteries is not very advanced, the arteries may be able to supply the needs of the heart at rest but not during exercise. Hence the ECG changes produced by deficient blood flow (ischaemia) may be seen only during exercise. In stress tests, exercise of measured and graded severity is performed under medical supervision. Therefore it is a much safer and better way of detecting transient changes in ECG than depending upon attacks of angina. Further, a stress test may detect the disease even before the patient has had any attacks of angina. Exercise during stress tests is provided through a stationary bicycle or a treadmill.

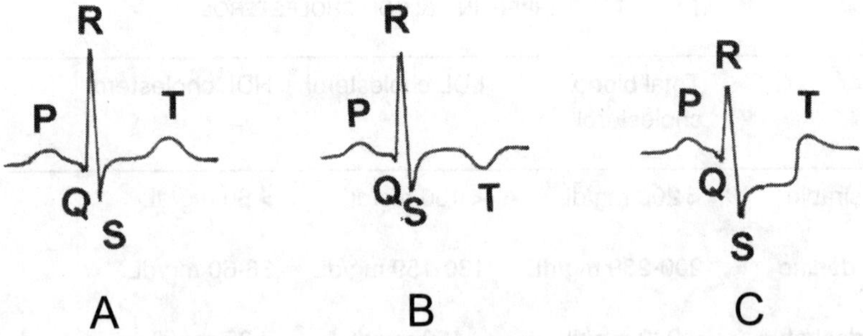

Fig. 10.5. *Electrocardiogram (ECG).*
A. Normal. B. & C. ECGs showing changes which may result from deficient blood supply to the heart.

The sensitivity of the stress test is increased if, during exercise, some of the following measurements are also made:
(a) Blood flow through the heart muscle using thallium 201,
(b) Ventricular volume and ejection fraction, using technetium 99 (ejection fraction is the percentage of the total volume of blood in the ventricle at the end of relaxation, which is pumped during contraction), or
(c) Movements of the heart, using echocardiography.

Angiography

During an angiography, material which is opaque to X-rays is injected into the coronary arteries. Therefore X-rays taken during the injection outline the inside of the coronary arteries. Hence the presence and degree of block in coronary arteries can be detected by an angiography.

RISK FACTORS FOR CAD

Several factors increase the probability of an individual getting CAD. These are called risk factors. Some of the risk factors, such as heredity, are non-modifiable; that is, we cannot do anything about them. It is more important to know the modifiable risk factors and do something about them.

> Do not worry about things which you can do nothing about.
> Do not worry about things which you can do something about: just do it.

Let us learn what the modifiable risk factors are, and what we can do about them.

1. Hyperlipidemia

High blood cholesterol level, specially LDL cholesterol level, is an established major risk factor for CAD. In contrast, HDL cholesterol is protective. An easy way to remember which cholesterol is good and which bad is to think of 'L for lousy; H for healthy'. Therefore a high HDL/LDL ratio is associated with a lower risk for CAD. Among Indians, high levels of blood triglycerides also seem to imply higher risk for CAD.

LDL and total cholesterol level in blood can be brought down by appropriate attention to diet and increase in physical activity. In addition, some drugs also lower blood cholesterol, and the newer drugs in this category are very effective. But drugs are advisable only if diet and exercise fail to achieve the desirable reduction in cholesterol level.

2. Smoking

Smoking is a major risk factor for CAD and several other cardiovascular diseases. Its predictive value for stroke and peripheral vascular disease (Buerger's disease) is even greater than for CAD.

Even after years of smoking, if one stops smoking, at least part of the damage already done can be reversed.

3. Hypertension

Hypertension (high blood pressure) is also a major risk factor for CAD. The relationship between hypertension and CAD has several facets:
- (a) Both may be due to a similar disease process: atherosclerosis.
- (b) Both have similar risk factors.
- (c) Hypertension, due to any cause, may lead to a CAD-like picture by imposing additional load on the heart.
- (d) Treating high blood pressure reduces mortality and morbidity due to the associated CAD.

4. Diabetes mellitus

Diabetes mellitus, and its much commoner precursor, impaired glucose tolerance (IGT), significantly increase the risk for CAD. Therefore prompt treatment of diabetes or IGT with proper diet and exercise, and if necessary, also drugs, helps in reducing the risk of CAD.

5. Obesity

Central obesity (ie obesity around the abdomen) is an independent risk factor for CAD. This type of obesity is specially common among Indians. In addition, simply being overweight is itself bad for CAD due to its associated features such as hyperlipidemia, hypertension and diabetes.

6. Physical activity

Sedentary life predisposes one to obesity, diabetes, hypertension and hyperlipidemia, which are risk factors for CAD. Correspondingly, physical activity reduces the risk of CAD. Physical activity is one of the most important measures directly under the control of the patient which have a significant impact on the onset and progress of CAD. Exercise also helps by encouraging the formation of collateral blood vessels (new interconnections) which can bypass at least part of the handicap produced by blocked arteries (Fig. 10.6).

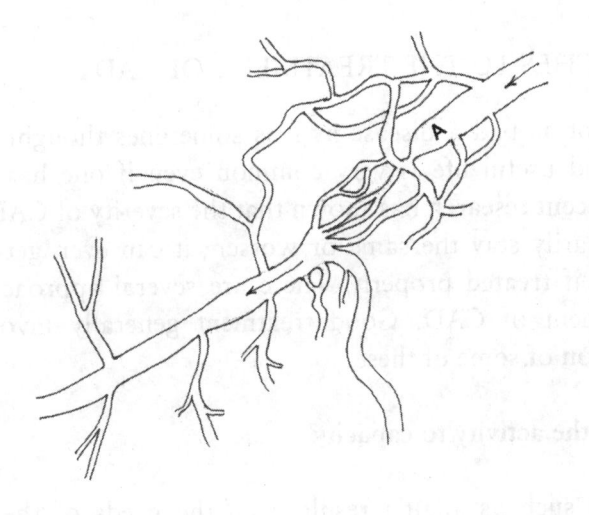

Fig. 10.6. *A diagrammatic sketch of a coronary angiogram showing how collateral blood vessels have neutralised the effect of a block at A.*

7. Mental stress

Mental stress, specially chronic stress resulting from certain personality characteristics is associated with increased risk of the onset and more rapid progress of CAD. It is commonly said that the personality which increases the susceptibility to CAD is the type A personality. Type A personality is characterised by high achievement orientation, a tendency towards multi-tasking (trying to do more than one thing at the same time), aggressiveness, jealousy, hostility, cynicism and competitiveness. However, all features of the type A personality are not related to

CAD. The features that actually increase the risk for CAD are aggressiveness, jealousy, hostility and cynicism. Thus hard work does not kill; nor do ambition, efficient time management and healthy competition by themselves lead to heart disease. It is the negative emotions that may be associated with type A personality that increase the risk for heart disease.

APPROACHES TO THE TREATMENT OF CAD

CAD is not as bad a disease as it is sometimes thought to be. A long and useful life is very common even if one has CAD. Further, recent research has shown that the severity of CAD does not necessarily stay the same or worsen; it can even get better with time if treated properly. There are several approaches to the treatment of CAD. Good treatment generally involves a combination of some of these.

Matching the activity to capacity

Symptoms such as angina result from the needs of the heart exceeding its capacity. Therefore symptoms can be prevented by avoiding situations in which the demands of the heart may exceed its capacity. This can be done by keeping the following in mind in one's daily life:

(a) The intensity and/or duration of physical activity should be reduced to a level that does not cause angina. For example, one may reduce the speed or distance during walking. If a certain distance has got to be walked for reaching the place of work, one can walk it slowly, and also have an interval of rest if necessary.

(b) Physical activity should be avoided at particular times, eg early morning and immediately after meals.

(c) The size of the meals should be reduced. To compensate for it, the number of meals per day may be increased, if necessary. Meals lead to an increase in blood flow through the stomach

and intestines, and thereby increase the work of the heart. The heavier the meal, the greater the increase in the workload of the heart.
(d) Emotional upheavals should be avoided. Anger releases adrenaline, which increases the rate and force of contraction of the heart. Sometimes one can feel the pounding of the heart in such situations. This increases the needs of the heart enormously, and the narrowed coronary arteries of a patient having CAD may not be able to meet these needs. The increase in the needs of the heart in emotional states may be far more than during physical exercise or after meals. Therefore, anger can prove to be more dangerous than physical exercise.

Lifestyle changes

The major components of lifestyle modification which are helpful in preventing and managing CAD have been discussed briefly below.

Smoking

Smoking is so harmful for the heart that it is important to stop it promptly and completely (Chapter 4).

Diet

The diet best suited for CAD (as well as for healthy people!) is a low fat, high fibre vegetarian diet (Chapter 3). Some practical tips for preparing such a diet are:
(a) Use minimal quantity of visible fat. The best oils to use are soyabean oil and mustard oil.
(b) Avoid eggs.
(c) Use unrefined cereals and pulses (i.e. with the husk intact)
(d) Eat plenty of vegetables and fruits – a total of about 400 g per day.

The quantity of the diet should be so adjusted as to attain and maintain normal body weight.

Besides what one eats, the yogic attitude of non-attachment to food helps in reducing stress, an important risk factor for CAD.

It is sometimes thought that the effect of the diet gets averaged out over a period of weeks or months, and therefore the composition of a single meal is not relevant. This is only partly true. Even a single heavy high-fat meal can precipitate a heart attack in a susceptible person by increasing the load on the heart on one hand (as discussed above), and reducing coronary blood flow by a variety of mechanisms on the other. That is why some people get a heart attack the night they return from a party, specially if they had also smoked and drank at the party.

Exercise

Keeping the degree of exercise within the limits imposed by the disease, one should lead a physically active life (Chapter 5). Exercise helps in several ways:
(a) It helps maintain normal body weight.
(b) It brings down blood cholesterol.
(c) It helps control concomitant diabetes, if present. If not present, exercise helps in reducing the risk of getting diabetes.
(d) It encourages the formation of collaterals (alternative channels for carrying blood to the heart).
(e) It reduces mental tension. This is specially true of yogic exercises, if performed with the right attitude. Incorporating some yogasanas in the daily routine and introducing a yogic attitude into even simple exercises like walking adds to their calming effect.

Stress management

The effect of emotional upheavals has already been outlined. Equally harmful is chronic stress variously manifesting as depression, worry or anxiety. It is common to blame our circumstances for stress. This is not entirely correct. Stress is the result of the interaction between the circumstances and the person. In fact, the reaction of the person to circumstances is much more important than the circumstances. This can be easily understood by observing people. Under very similar circumstances, one person may be miserable and another cheerful. Further, changing the circumstances does not guarantee happiness. A person who, by nature, is the worrying type, will find new reasons for worry in the new circumstances. Yoga helps in inculcating an attitude which ensures calm and peace in all circumstances (Chapter 7).

Controlling associated conditions

Conditions such as obesity, high blood pressure and diabetes, which are frequently present together with CAD should be controlled. Their interactions are such that, if not properly controlled, they make CAD get worse. On the other hand, most of the measures outlined above help also these associated conditions. For high blood pressure, restricting salt in the diet is likely to help. Further, drugs may be necessary to control high blood pressure and diabetes.

Drugs

The type of drugs commonly used for CAD, and their rationale, are briefly given below.

Nitrates

Nitroglycerine and Sorbitrate are the common drugs of this category. They act by relaxing the walls of coronary arteries, thereby making them wider. However, they do not remove the fatty deposits which block the arteries. Therefore the effect of these drugs lasts only for a few hours. However, these drugs are valuable for prompt relief of angina, as well as for prevention of angina if taken in anticipation. The tablet is usually kept under the tongue. It should ideally be used whenever exertion which is likely to produce angina is undertaken. If not taken before hand, the next best is to keep the tablet under the tongue as soon after angina as possible.

Tolerance to nitrates develops with continuous use, which makes them ineffective. Therefore a minimum of eight hours at a stretch per day should be spent without these drugs for them to remain effective.

Nitroglycerine is inactivated by exposure to moisture, air and sunlight. If the tablets seem to have become ineffective (i.e. when they neither relieve pain of angina nor bring on the headache, which is their side effect), they should be discarded.

It is useful to maintain a daily record of the time at which each tablet is used. It helps you as well as your doctor in monitoring the disease.

Beta blockers

These drugs block the effect of adrenaline on the heart and many other parts of the body. Adrenaline is released during anger and exercise. Thus beta blockers do not allow adrenaline to raise the heart rate during such states. However, adrenaline acts not only on the heart but also at several other places. Beta blockers do not let adrenaline act at some of these other places also: that may give side effects. But in spite of the side effects, beta blockers are useful for several patients.

Calcium antagonists

Contraction of the heart as well as other muscles of the body depends on very small quantities of calcium leaking into them during activation. Calcium antagonists reduce this leak into the heart as well as the muscular lining of coronary arteries and other blood vessels of the body. Reducing calcium entry into the heart reduces the contractility of the heart and thereby reduces its work load, specially during exercise or anger. Reducing calcium entry into coronary arteries prevents their contraction, or in other words, opens them up (i.e. dilates them). Reducing calcium entry into other arteries of the body dilates these too, and thereby brings down the blood pressure. Reducing the blood pressure also reduces the work load of the heart. That is why calcium antagonists also help several patients having CAD. However, their side effects and interactions with beta blockers make their use limited and complicated.

Aspirin

Aspirin in low doses has been used extensively for several decades now for its tendency to prevent clot formation. Theoretically that should prevent a heart attack by reducing the possibility of a clot forming in a partially blocked coronary artery and blocking it completely rather suddenly. Studies do support this expectation, but whether preventing clot formation is completely desirable from every angle is doubtful. For example, reduced tendency of the blood to clot could be deleterious in case of a stroke due to brain hemorrhage (bleeding).

Lipid lowering drugs

Lipid lowering drugs are used only if lifestyle modification has failed to lower total and LDL cholesterol levels. In that case, the diet control is made stricter and a drug or combination of drugs is also added to the treatment. The most commonly used drugs in this category are the statins. However, drugs have side effects, and therefore their use and dosage should be monitored by a doctor.

Angioplasty (PTCA) and related procedures

PTCA stands for Percutaneous Transluminal Coronary Angioplasty. In this procedure a tiny balloon is advanced to the site of the block with the help of a guidewire. The balloon is introduced in a deflated state, but when it reaches the block, it is inflated. Then the wire and balloon are removed, but much of the effect of inflation stays for some time. However, with time the block may recur. Several modifications of angioplasty are aimed at preventing the recurrence. One approach is to implant a stent in the artery at the site of the block. A stent is a metallic device to hold the artery wide open. Unlike the balloon, which is pulled out, the stent is left in the blocked artery. Another approach is to reach the blocked artery in the same way as in angioplasty, and then to try to remove or crush the plaque by using laser or some mechanical device.

None of the above procedures guarantees that there will be no recurrence of symptoms. Symptoms may recur due to a block at the same place or some other place in the coronary arteries. Therefore lifestyle modification is important even after angioplasty or any other related procedure, and offers the best hope for the longest symptom-free period.

Bypass surgery (CABG)

CABG stands for coronary artery bypass grafting. As the name indicates, the procedure bypasses the block. Two types of procedure are common for creating the bypass (Fig. 10.7). In one,

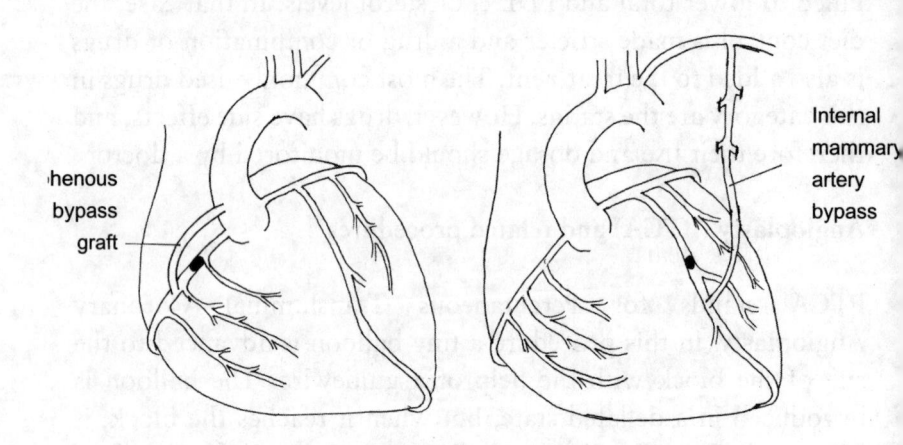

Fig. 10.7. *A diagrammatic representation of two types of bypass surgery. The blocks in the coronary arteries which have been bypassed have also been indicated.*

a piece of saphenous vein (a vein in the leg) is grafted between the aorta (the biggest artery arising from the heart) and a site on the diseased coronary artery beyond the block. In the other, an artery in the chest (the internal mammary artery) is joined to a site on the affected coronary artery beyond the block.

Bypass surgery provides a solution which generally lasts longer than angioplasty. But, with time, the bypass may also be affected by the same disease process which led to CAD. Therefore lifestyle modification is important even after a bypass surgery to prevent recurrence of symptoms.

Frequently Asked Questions

1. *What is meant by (a) ischaemia, (b) angina, and (c) atherosclerosis?*

    (a) Ischaemia is deficient blood supply to an organ. If coronary arteries are blocked, the heart suffers from ischaemia. That is why coronary artery disease (CAD) or coronary heart disease (CHD) is also called ischaemic heart disease (IHD).
    (b) Angina is the typical discomfort in chest as seen in CAD.
    (c) Atherosclerosis is the deposition of fatty substances in arteries. It is a generalised process affecting arteries throughout the body. But its effects are felt the most in:
    (i) the heart, where it leads to CAD,
    (ii) the brain, where it may lead to a stroke,
    (iii) the kidneys, where it may lead to renal hypertension and chronic renal failure, and
    (iv) the legs, where it leads to pain while walking.

2. *What is the effect of hydrogenated oils on blood cholesterol?*

    Vegetable oils, when hydrogenated, become saturated. Further, saturated fatty acids in hydrogenated oils are trans-fatty acids, which are worse than the naturally occurring saturated fatty acids in animal fats. Hydrogenated oils not only raise LDL cholesterol, they also lower HDL cholesterol, which makes them doubly harmful.

3. *Do nuts contain cholesterol, and can those having CAD take them?*

   Nuts do not contain cholesterol. In fact, no vegetable food contains any cholesterol. However, nuts do contain a large amount of fat. But this fat is largely unsaturated fat, and therefore has a tendency to lower blood cholesterol. Therefore those having CAD can have nuts. The only precaution necessary is that the total energy intake should not exceed requirements. Hence the energy obtained from nuts should be compensated by reducing the quantity of some other food. The goal is to maintain normal body weight (also see Chapter 3).

4. *What is Lp(a)?*

   Lp(a) is a lipoprotein closely related to LDL. High levels of Lp(a) also increase the risk for CAD. The levels of Lp(a) are largely determined by the genetic make up of the individual. Dietary changes which lower total and LDL cholesterol do not affect the level of Lp(a) in blood.

5. *What is homocysteine?*

   Homocysteine is an amino acid. (Amino acids are building blocks of proteins). There is some evidence that high levels of homocysteine in the blood increase the risk for CAD. Deficiency of folic acid (a B-vitamin, found in green leafy vegetables) leads to high homocysteine levels. Therefore, to avoid this risk factor, one should consume plenty of green leafy vegetables.

6. *How long after angioplasty or a bypass surgery, can a person join a lifestyle modification course?*

   As a rule of the thumb, after three months. This applies only to the yogic postures or other forms of exercise. Changes in diet, managing stress, and stopping smoking do not have to wait: these lifestyle modifications may be started immediately after the intervention – the sooner the better. However, since the major component of most lifestyle modification courses is physical activity, joining a formal course may be delayed by three months. Finally, before joining such a course, it is important to get the approval of your cardiologist.

11

Too Sweet

Sweet are the uses of adversity.
                                    WILLIAM SHAKESPEARE

Diabetes is a common disease which is getting commoner at an alarming rate. In Indian cities, at least one out of every ten adults has diabetes. The villages are relatively spared, where the ratio is about one for every thirty. The disease develops so slowly and silently that only half of those who have diabetes know that they have it. Further, there are apparently healthy people, just as many as those with diabetes, who will get diabetes in a few years unless they make significant changes in their lifestyle. This forecast can be made available to these people (technically, having impaired glucose tolerance, or IGT) on the basis of a simple blood test. On the brighter side, the management of diabetes has now advanced to a point where a diabetic can hope to live just as long and productive a life as a non-diabetic, provided he understands his problem and participates actively in his own treatment. Understanding the problem is desirable in all diseases, but in case of diabetes it is absolutely essential. In order to participate actively in taking care of the illness, the patient along with his family should also understand the illness. Managing diabetes properly does not mean living a dull and monotonous life. The life of a diabetic need be hardly different from that of a sensible and balanced non-diabetic.

WHAT HAPPENS IN DIABETES?

What is commonly called diabetes is more accurately termed diabetes mellitus (DM). DM is a disorder resulting from the deficiency of the hormone called insulin – absolute or relative. Absolute deficiency means that the body produces less insulin. Relative deficiency means that although insulin is available, it is unable to act. Relative deficiency is also called insulin resistance (IR), which means that the body is resistant to the actions of insulin.

Insulin is produced by the pancreas (Fig. 11.1). The pancreas is an organ which produces two types of chemicals. To one category belong some of the most important enzymes required for the digestion of food. To the other category belong a few hormones, one of which is insulin. Insulin is produced by the B cells of the pancreas.

About ninety per cent of those who have diabetes have type 2 diabetes. In type 1 diabetes, there is a rather severe absolute deficiency of insulin. In type 2 diabetes, the predominant defect is insulin resistance. Type 2 diabetes has also been called NIDDM (non-insulin dependent diabetes mellitus) and maturity onset diabetes. But currently the preferred term is type 2 diabetes because the other two terms are misleading. NIDDM is misleading because many patients having type 2 diabetes have to be treated with insulin after they have had the disease for a few years. Maturity onset diabetes is misleading because many persons with type 2 diabetes are quite young; in fact, there is a trend towards developing the disorder at a younger age.

Why is insulin so important?

Insulin plays a key role in the proper utilisation of the major nutrients: carbohydrates, proteins and fats. Nutrients have two

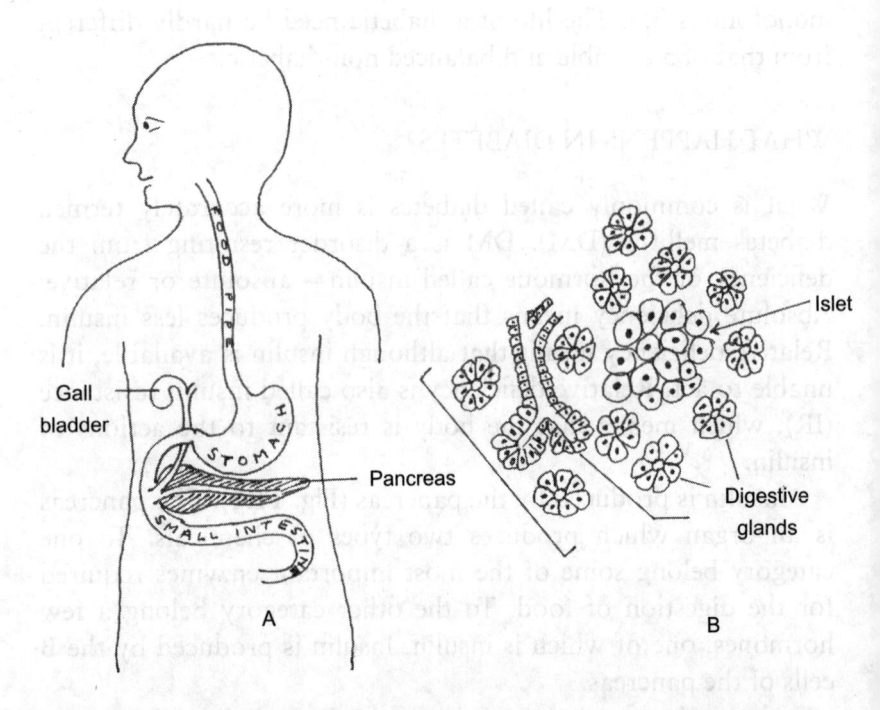

Fig. 11.1. A. *The pancreas sits snugly in the arms of the C-shaped part of the small intestine.*
B. *A diagrammatic sketch of a very thin slice of the pancreas, as seen under a microscope. The pancreas is a two-in-one organ. Most of it has glands which manufacture a digestive juice. The juice reaches the small intestine through a narrow tube (shown in A). But interspersed between digestive glands are also islands having a very different type of cells. These islands, called islets, have B cells which secrete insulin, and also cells which secrete some other hormones.*

major functions: to supply energy, and to supply the material for repair of wear and tear. To these may be added a third function: to favour the storage of nutrients which can be mobilised in times of scarcity. Insulin is required for each of these functions. It is required for utilisation of glucose, the key nutrient which supplies energy. It is required for the synthesis of proteins, the building blocks for growth and repair and also for the synthesis of triglycerides, the form in which fats are stored in the body.

What happens in the case of insulin deficiency?

If the body cannot manufacture enough insulin, or insulin cannot act due to insulin resistance, the net result in either case is that the body suffers from insulin deficiency.

Since insulin is required for utilisation of glucose, its deficiency leads to inadequate utilisation. The result is that the glucose derived from food stays under-utilised in the body. Hence it accumulates in the body, and that leads to a higher concentration of glucose in the blood (hyperglycemia). Thus the blood is literally flooded with glucose but the body is starved for the want of fuel. The paradox has been summed up in the expression 'starvation in the midst of plenty'.

As in starvation, a person having diabetes feels hungry. Therefore he eats a lot. Further, as in starvation, the body also mobilises its reserves. On the other hand, deficient action of insulin means that the reserves cannot be built up. Hence, in spite of eating a lot, the person loses weight.

Since the blood glucose level is high, some of the glucose spills over in the urine. To be more precise, whenever the blood glucose is above 180mg/dL, glucose can be detected in the urine (Fig. 11.2).

Since glucose in the urine has to be dissolved in water, more urine has to be passed for the sake of excreting glucose. Hence the total volume of urine passed per day goes up.

Since more water is lost from the body in the form of urine, the loss has to be made up by drinking water. Hence the person drinks a lot of water.

We have discussed above the mechanisms underlying some of the well-known features of diabetes: high blood glucose (hyperglycemia), eating too much (polyphagia), loss of weight, glucose in the urine (glucosuria), frequent urination (polyuria), and excessive thirst (polydipsia).

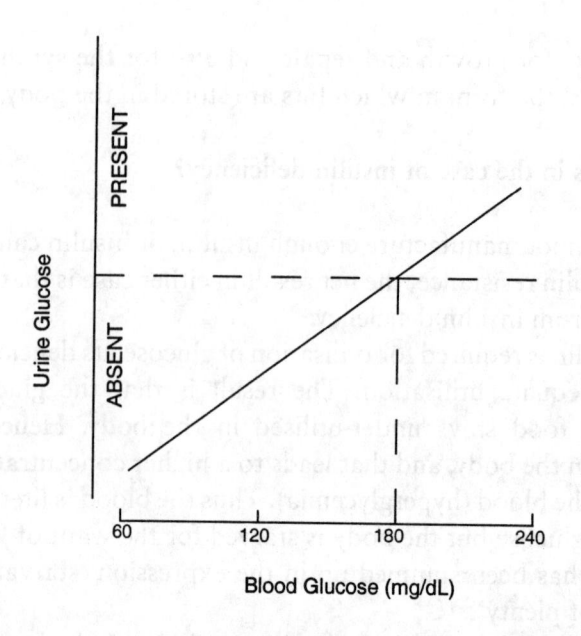

Fig.11.2. *So long as the blood glucose is below 180 mg/dL, glucose does not appear in the urine. With blood glucose values above 180 mg/dL, glucose is present in urine: higher the blood glucose, higher is the concentration of glucose in the urine.*

SYMPTOMS OF DIABETES

The classical symptoms of diabetes are loss of weight (in spite of eating rather well), frequent urination and excessive thirst. But if these symptoms develop slowly, and are not very severe, they are not alarming. Moreover, in mild or moderate cases, these symptoms may not be there at all. That is why diabetes may remain undetected for years unless a urine or blood test reveals it unexpectedly. Sometimes diabetes is first diagnosed when the patient has repeated infections, an ulcer which refuses to heal, or a persistent itch or rash over the skin. These are signals for a doctor to suspect diabetes. In some cases, diabetes may be first detected through its complications, some of which have been discussed below.

COMPLICATIONS OF DIABETES

With diabetes having become treatable, the lifespan of a diabetic is essentially normal. But unless the patient is meticulous in following the treatment, complications of diabetes do occur, and are a major cause of death and disability. The three major complications of diabetes are retinopathy, neuropathy and nephropathy.

Retinopathy

Retinopathy refers to an abnormality in the retina. The retina is the 'screen' in the eyes on which the 'picture' of whatever is seen is first projected. The earliest stage of diabetic retinopathy is symptomless, but can be detected by an examination of the eye. If enough precautions are taken at this stage, the progress to serious sight-threatening stages can be largely prevented. Therefore, an annual check-up of the eyes is a must for a person having diabetes.

Nephropathy

Nephropathy refers to an abnormality in the kidneys. Nephropathy is also one of the complications predictably and consistently associated with the duration and quality of control of diabetes. If a person has hypertension, or has a family history of hypertension, it adds to the risk of developing diabetic nephropathy. Invariably, retinopathy occurs before nephropathy. Once again, prevention is better and easier than cure and of an annual urine examination for microalbuminaria is a must for a person having diabetes.

Neuropathy

Neuropathy refers to an abnormality of the nerves. Neuropathy is an early and almost universal complication of diabetes, but it is symptomless in the majority. If symptoms do occur, they can have a wide range because nerves are there all over the body. The symptoms include weakness, inability to feel stimuli applied to the skin, indigestion, constipation or diarrhoea, poor control of the urinary bladder, excessive sweating, or a tendency to faint while getting up.

Diabetic foot

Ulceration of the foot, which resists healing, is a common complication of diabetes. It should not be taken lightly because it may eventually make amputation of the leg necessary.

A diabetic foot develops due to contributions from other complications of diabetes. Neuropathy makes injuries to the foot painless, leading to their neglect. Insufficient blood supply to the legs and feet, which is a common feature of diabetes, delays healing. Delayed healing promotes infection of the wound. The infection delays healing further, thus setting up a vicious cycle.

Hypertension and Coronary Artery Disease

Although these diseases can occur quite independently of diabetes, there are enough linkages to make hypertension, coronary artery disease and diabetes occur as a cluster in the same person. Further, diabetes adds to the risk of developing hypertension and coronary artery disease. It is also good to keep in mind that, due to neuropathy, the chest pain of heart disease may not be felt by a person having diabetes. Hence the person may have heart disease but remain unaware of it till it is quite advanced.

Prevention of complications

There is enough evidence to state emphatically that complications are directly related to the degree and duration of hyperglycemia. Hence the complications can be largely prevented by controlling diabetes properly. Complications occur the least if glycated haemoglobin level is maintained close to seven per cent (see below). While the prevention of complications is feasible, reversing them is almost impossible. Once a complication such as retinopathy or nephropathy has occurred, the best that can be done is to slow down its rate of further progress.

LABORATORY TESTS IN DIABETES

The laboratory tests commonly performed for detecting diabetes and for monitoring its control and progress have been described briefly below. However, the emphasis is on tests suitable for monitoring the control of diabetes because those are the tests the patient has to undergo. Tests for detecting or diagnosing diabetes are ordered by the doctor and done in a laboratory.

Urine

The urine is generally examined for the presence of glucose and protein.

Glucose

The kidney normally filters glucose but then takes it back into the circulation completely. Therefore there is no glucose in the urine. However, if the level of blood glucose is high, the level of glucose in the renal filtrate is also high. And there is a limit to which the kidney can take glucose back into the circulation. Therefore any glucose that is left behind in the filtrate, after the kidney has returned back to the circulation as much glucose as it can, appears in the urine.

Glucose generally appears in the urine if the blood glucose level is above 180 mg/dL (Fig. 11.2). In a healthy person the blood glucose never crosses this limit, but in a person having diabetes it might, particularly after a meal. Therefore, it is best to examine a urine sample collected one to two hours after a meal to detect diabetes at an early stage.

Protein

The kidney normally does not filter protein. But if the kidney has been damaged, as a complication of diabetes or hypertension or otherwise, protein is filtered, and the filtered protein can be detected in the urine.

Blood

Blood is commonly examined for glucose to detect or monitor diabetes but a few other tests may also be done sometimes.

Glucose

Blood glucose is the commonest and most reliable test for detecting diabetes. As may be deduced from the above discussion on urine glucose, blood glucose may be above normal, but so long as it is below 180 mg/dL, glucose will not appear in the urine. Therefore mild diabetes can be detected only though the blood glucose test.

Random blood glucose

If the blood sample is collected without any consideration of when the last meal was taken, it is called a random sample. Random blood glucose is the least reliable for diagnosing diabetes, but is frequently done for the sake of convenience. If the random blood glucose is above 200 mg/dL, especially if it is associated with one of the symptoms of diabetes, it is enough to diagnose diabetes. Even a random blood glucose of above 125 mg/dL warrants further investigation through more reliable tests.

Fasting blood glucose

If the blood sample is collected at least eight hours after the last meal, it is called a fasting sample. Fasting blood glucose should ideally be less than 110 mg/dL. The range from 110-125 mg/dL is suspicious, and these days is called 'impaired fasting glucose'.

Postprandial blood glucose

Postprandial (PP) blood glucose is done on a sample collected 2 hours after a meal: it should be less than 200 mg/dL. PP glucose is a valuable tool for monitoring diabetes. Its value depends not only on the health status of the individual but also on the type of meal taken.

Oral glucose tolerance test

An oral glucose tolerance test (OGTT) is done by giving 75g glucose to a person after an overnight fast. In addition to a fasting blood sample, another sample is collected two hours after giving the glucose. OGTT is a valuable tool for diagnosing diabetes (Table 1).

TABLE 1. DIAGNOSTIC CRITERIA PROPOSED BY THE AMERICAN DIABETES ASSOCIATION (2000)

	FPG (mg/dL)	2-h PG (mg/dL)
Normal	< 110	< 140
Impaired fasting glucose	110-125	
Impaired glucose tolerance		140-199
Diabetes mellitus	≥ 126	≥ 200

FPG, fasting plasma glucose; 2-h PG, plasma glucose 2h after taking 75g glucose

Glycated haemoglobin

Glycated (or glycosylated) haemoglobin, abbreviated as HbA_1C, is formed in blood as the result of a small fraction of haemoglobin reacting with glucose. The higher the glucose level, the greater the amount of this transformed haemoglobin. Glycated haemoglobin level gives an overall picture of blood glucose over the preceding three months, particularly the preceding one month. Since complications of diabetes are closely related to the overall maintenance of blood glucose, one of the aims of good management of diabetes is to maintain the glycated haemoglobin level at about seven per cent.

Blood lipids

Blood cholesterol, and its fractions (LDL and HDL) are also indicators of the quality of control in diabetes. For some details about blood lipids, please consult the IHC booklet on coronary artery disease.

TREATMENT

Diet, exercise and medication have been the three traditional pillars in the treatment of diabetes. To these may be added lifestyle measures other than diet and exercise, and patient education.

Diet

The current opinion about the dietary management of diabetes is full of good news. The diet of a diabetic can now be a reasonably normal, healthy and palatable diet. In fact, the diet recommended for a diabetic is one which everybody else should also take to prevent diabetes and several other diseases. For Indians, there is further good news that the diet which is healthy for all is essentially the traditional Indian vegetarian diet. With this background, let us see what the current recommendations are regarding diet in case of diabetes.

Energy

If a person having diabetes is overweight, his total food intake should be restricted. In such cases, it is better to consume about 500 kcal less than the energy requirement. This degree of restriction generally achieves a weight loss of about half a kilogram a week. After desirable body weight has been achieved, the energy intake should match the energy requirement. An overweight person is likely to achieve an improvement in glucose tolerance just by losing some weight. A mildly diabetic person may get cured just by losing a few kilos.

As a rule of the thumb, the desirable body weight in kg is equal to the height in cm minus 100. A diabetic should try to maintain a weight which is further ten per cent less. Thus a 160 cm tall diabetic should aim at a weight of 54 kg (160 − 100 = 60 kg, 60 − 10% of 60 = 60 − 6 = 54 kg).

Carbohydrates

Carbohydrates make up the single largest constituent of the diet, and are just as important for a diabetic as anybody else. The diabetics can take about seventy per cent of their energy intake in the form of carbohydrates, which is the norm in a good Indian diet.

The intestines digest carbohydrates into glucose and related substances. Therefore the blood level of glucose goes up after a meal. However, all carbohydrates do not push up the blood glucose level to the same extent. The aim of diabetic diets (and in any healthy diet) is to have foods which push up the blood glucose level as little as possible. Such foods are said to have a low glycemic index (GI). Further, we generally do not take single foods but mixed meals. Therefore what is important is to take low GI meals.

The GI of a meal gives the immediate impact of a food on the blood glucose level. Another important consideration is the long-term impact of the food on glucose tolerance. Fortunately foods which have a low GI also improve glucose tolerance. Let us now see what type of carbohydrate-rich foods are able to achieve both these aims.

1. Complex carbohydrates are better than simple carbohydrates. Starch is a complex carbohydrate. Starch is found in cereals, pulses, bananas, potatoes, etc. Sugar is a simple carbohydrate, and has a high GI.
2. Although sugar has a high GI, as discussed earlier, it is the GI of the meal which is important. A small amount of sugar has very little impact on the GI of an otherwise low-GI meal. In short, sugar should be in good company. Constituents of the diet which are particularly good at blunting the GI of meals are:
   (a) fibre, available from whole grains, fruits and vegetables,
   (b) proteins, specially abundant in pulses, milk and meat,
   (c) fats

Since Indians generally have tea with milk, the tea has in it an in-built constituent for reducing GI. Further, if a biscuit or some snack is taken with tea, it will further blunt the effect of sugar. However, in the pursuit of a low GI, one should not make the tea very heavy because first, the glycemic response depends not only on what the meal contains but also on the total quantity of food in the meal. Secondly, GI is not the only thing to think about: we also have to keep the daily energy intake at the desirable level.

Indian sweets also generally have sugar. In short, in moderation, sweetened tea or sweets are quite acceptable for a diabetic. As a rule of the thumb, it has been recommended that in a diabetic diet not more than ten per cent of the energy intake should come from sugar. That gives an adult diabetic permission to take a maximum of 8 teaspoonfuls of sugar, provided the principles discussed above are kept in mind, and the total energy intake is within the prescribed limit. If keeping so many things in mind is difficult, it is better not to take sugar. Not taking sugar does no harm to anybody, whether or not a person has diabetes.

3. Whole grains have a lower GI than refined (dehusked) grains, because of the difference in fibre content. Therefore atta is preferable to maida, brown rice is better than white rice, brown bread is better than white bread, and whole (*sabut*) dals are better than refined (*dhuli*) dals.
4. Fermented foods, eg idlis, have a lower GI than an unfermented food having the same constituents.
5. Unripe bananas have a lower GI than ripe bananas.
6. Cooked dals, rice or potato which have been stored in the refrigerator have a lower GI than freshly cooked foods, even if the refrigerated foods are heated before eating.

In short, carbohydrates in the diet should come primarily from whole grains (cereals and pulses). Although, with some precautions, sugar is acceptable in moderation, it is best avoided.

Fats

In the context of Indian diets, fats should provide 15-20 per cent of the energy intake. Since some fat comes from grains (invisible fat), a person may take an additional 20-30g fat per day in visible form, preferably through a judicious combination of fats. If a single source of fat has to be chosen as the cooking medium, mustard oil or soyabean oil is the best choice. (Please see Chapter 3 for more details).

Proteins

Proteins should provide 10-15 per cent of the energy intake. An adequate quantity of protein of satisfactory quality may be obtained from a diet based primarily on a combination of cereals and pulses.

Vitamins, minerals and antioxidants

Good sources of these nutrients are vegetables, specially green leafy vegetables, fruits and spices. Adequate intake may be achieved by taking five helpings of fruits/vegetables (total about 400g) per day, and moderate quantities of herbs and spices, such as onions, garlic, ginger, lemon, cinnamon, tejpatta, curry leaves, tulsi and pepper. Fenugreek seeds have been found to be particularly beneficial for diabetes. The recommended dose is 25-50g per day depending on the severity of diabetes. Although the seeds are bitter, if added while making chapattis, rice, dal and vegetables, the food tastes quite aright.

Alcohol

Although alcohol is, strictly speaking, not a food, it may be discussed here because it is consumed like food. Alcohol carries for diabetics on medication the special risk of inducing hypoglycemia (low blood sugar). In addition, those taking chlorpropamide for diabetes get flushing, nausea and dizziness. Alcohol also increases the risk of cataract, and that of high levels of blood triglycerides. Therefore besides all the reasons for which anybody should avoid alcohol, those having diabetes have additional reasons to do so. However, if one must, the diabetic should consume a maximum of 28 g of alcohol per day (about 50 ml of whiskey or 500 ml of beer), drink it slowly, and with food. Wine, specially red wine, has earned a good reputation because it contains some antioxidants. But there are so many alternative sources of antioxidants that this fact need not be used as an excuse for consuming alcohol.

If a person consumes alcohol, its contribution to energy intake should be taken into account since it provides 7 kcal/g. For purposes of calculation, the energy derived from alcohol should be treated as if it came from fats.

Meal pattern

Insulin is required for utilising food, and in a diabetic who is not on medication, the insulin stock is low. Therefore the meal should be such that it should need less insulin. This requirement is met easily by keeping two things in mind: first, it should be a small meal; and second, it should be a low GI meal. If each meal is small, and still the nutritional needs have to be fulfilled, the number of meals should be increased. Hence the person should take small and frequent meals. This is a good arrangement even if the diabetic is not on medication. However, if he is on medication, additional care is required to ensure that when the action of insulin or a hypoglycemic tablet is on, food should be available. If food is not available, the insulin or tablet may take the blood glucose down to a dangerously low level. To avoid such accidents, the diabetic on medication should not miss a meal, and should observe reasonable constancy in the timing and quantity of meals.

A sample distribution of energy intake based on six meals is as follows:

Breakfast 15%, mid-morning 5%, lunch 35%, evening 5%, dinner 30%, bedtime 10%. A sample diet chart for a diabetic who should take 2000 kcal/day is given in Table 2.

TABLE 2. A 2000-KCAL DIABETIC DIET

	Carbohydrate (g)	Protein (g)	Fat (g)	Energy (kcal)
Breakfast	45	11	9	300
Brown bread: 2 slices				
Fruit: 1 helping				
Milk: 1 cup with				
1 spoon of sugar				
Mid-morning	15	1.5	3	90
Biscuit: One (about 20g)				
Tea: 1 cup with				
1 spoon of sugar				
Lunch	125	22	12	700
Chapattis: 2 (about 25g each)				
Rice: 1 helping (about 40g)				
Dal, sabut: 1 helping (about 50g)				
Vegetable: 1 helping (about 100g)				
Salad: about 100g				
Evening	25	1.5	1	115
Banana: One, small				
Tea: 1 cup with				
1 spoon sugar				
Dinner	112	22	9	610
Chapattis: 3 (about 25g each)				
Dal, sabut: 1 helping (about 50g)				
Vegetable: 1 helping (about 100g)				
Salad: about 100g				
Bedtime	30	3	8	200
Biscuits: 3 (about 20g each)				
TOTAL	352 g	61 g	42 g	2015 kcal
Contribution to energy	70%	12%	18%	

Scientific opinion about the diet suitable in case of diabetes has undergone revolutionary changes within the last few decades. The latest understanding of the subject allows an essentially normal prudent diet. Thus neither is the patient denied any reasonable food, nor does the family have to go through the inconvenience of providing a special diet to the patient. The few guidelines to be followed may be viewed as a boon in the sense that the entire family would get a healthy diet if it eats the same food as the patient. The diet which is good for managing diabetes is also good for preventing obesity, diabetes and cardiovascular diseases. The only additional care required in diabetes is that the meals should be relatively constant in quantity and timing, and no meal should be missed, specially if the patient is on medication.

Exercise

Exercise is an essential part of the treatment of diabetes. Exercise uses up glucose and improves the sensitivity of the body to insulin. In addition, it also helps in losing weight and preventing heart disease and high blood pressure. However, exercise uses up glucose. Therefore it has a tendency to reduce the level of blood glucose. To prevent the accidental fall of blood glucose to a dangerously low level, exercise, also like the diet, has to be regular and constant. Some sugar should be kept handy during exercise so that it can be eaten at the earliest sign of low blood glucose. On the other hand, if exercise is missed on some day, it is desirable to compensate for it by eating less at the meal next to the scheduled time for exercise.

However, before commencing upon any regime of vigorous exercises, it is important to make sure that the heart is healthy, and that there is no sign of retinopathy. Certain yogic postures can also be harmful in these situations. These precautions are particularly important in elderly diabetics.

Medication

In mild cases of type 2 diabetes, diet control and exercise may be enough to achieve normal blood glucose. However, if these measures prove inadequate, medication is required. Even when medication is used, diet control and exercise should continue. Medication may be in the form of either insulin injections or oral hypoglycemic agents (OHA) given as tablets.

Insulin

Since insulin has to be injected, it is generally not the preferred treatment. However, as initial therapy, insulin has a place even in case of type 2 diabetes. After a few weeks, the patient can generally be shifted from insulin to OHA.

Insulin may also be required in patients who have been having type 2 diabetes for several years and have been controlled satisfactorily with OHA. As the years pass, the capacity of the pancreas to secrete insulin may deteriorate, or insulin resistance may increase. In such situations also, insulin has to be used, either alone or in combination with OHA.

In type 1 diabetes, the body loses almost all its capacity to manufacture insulin. Therefore insulin injections are the only medication suitable for type 1 diabetes.

<u>Injecting insulin</u>

Insulin has to be injected just under the skin (subcutaneous or s.c.), which is easier than the more familiar intramuscular (i.m.) injection. And, since the injection is required at least once a day, the patient or a member of his family should be able to give it; it is not very practical to depend on a doctor or nurse. With care and practice, the technique of injection can be learnt easily.

The injection is commonly given with a disposable plastic syringe or a disposable 'pen' device. After assembling at one place the injection device, insulin, alcohol (spirit) and cotton, hands should be washed clean with soap and water. The insulin is drawn into the syringe. The skin at the site of injection is cleaned with spirit. The common sites are the tummy, upper arms, outer thighs and buttocks. Allow the spirit to dry. Stretch the skin and pinch it up with the left hand to make a skin fold. Hold the syringe like a pencil with the right hand. Pierce the skin with the needle at an angle of about 90°. Try to withdraw the plunger of the syringe. If blood enters the syringe, do not inject the insulin: change the site of injection. If no blood enters the syringe, inject insulin. Before withdrawing the needle, hold a cotton swab soaked in spirit near the needle. As soon as the needle is out, press the site of injection with the cotton swab. The next injection should be at a different site.

Oral hypoglycaemic agents

As tablets are more convenient than injections, OHA are the preferred medication in case of type 2 diabetes, whenever feasible. Most of the tablets currently in use have a duration of action of twelve to twenty four hours. Therefore the tablets have to be taken once or twice a day. In most cases, it is appropriate to take the dose thirty minutes before a principal meal. Since their duration of action is up to twenty four hours, it is unsafe to miss a meal scheduled even twelve hours after taking the tablet: missing the meal might lead to a dangerously low level of blood glucose.

Other than the tripod

Diet, exercise and medication constitute the tripod on which management of diabetes rests. But since diabetes is a condition needing lifelong care, and the patient's participation in his own treatment is extremely important, knowledge about several other management-related issues is vital.

Self-monitoring of blood glucose

Every diabetic on medication should assess how well his diabetes is controlled by measuring the blood glucose level at least once a day. The aim of the measurement is to make sure that the elevations in blood glucose due to meals, and the drops due to insulin or OHA, are not too big. Monitoring of blood glucose is required more frequently in patients on insulin than in those on OHA. The patient can himself measure blood glucose by using special chemically coated strips. A rough idea of blood glucose may be had by examining the strip visually, but for a more accurate measurement a glucometer is required. Several brands of relatively inexpensive user-friendly glucometers are available in the market.

Identifying and managing hypoglycemia

Nature releases insulin from the pancreas whenever required at exactly the right time and in the right amount. In diabetes, we try to mimic nature by giving either insulin or OHA, or sometimes both. But we are not perfect, and therefore sometimes the action of insulin or OHA brings the blood glucose down to levels below normal. The condition in which blood glucose level is below normal is called hypoglycemia. Severe hypoglycemia is a dangerous condition because the brain ordinarily uses only glucose as fuel. Therefore, if severe hypoglycemia persists for long, it can lead to unconsciousness, and even death.

Causes of hypoglycemia

In a person having diabetes and taking insulin or OHA for treatment, hypoglycemia may result from:
1. missing or delaying a meal, or taking a smaller meal than usual,
2. exercise, which is heavier than usual, or at an unusual time,
3. an overdose of insulin or OHA,
4. alcohol, or
5. intensification of treatment. If a patient starts taking additional exercise, becomes more careful with the quantity and quality of meals, loses weight, and brings down the level of mental stress – all without any reduction in the dose of insulin or OHA, the person may go into hypoglycemia.

Symptoms

It is important for the patient and his family to be able to identify hypoglycemia from its early manifestations so that they can take remedial action in time. The early manifestations include palpitation, sweating, hunger, a feeling of anxiety or irritability, and inability to concentrate. As hypoglycemia worsens, the patient may behave in a confusing manner, speaking may become difficult, there may be muscular incoordination, nausea and headache, and finally the person may become unconscious.

Although severe hyperglycemia (high blood glucose) may also be sometimes associated with loss of consciousness, when in doubt, it is safer to treat unconsciousness in a diabetic as if it was due to hypoglycemia.

Prevention

The prevention of hypoglycemia is not only better but also easier and safer than its cure. One has to basically understand that blood glucose should neither be too low nor too high. To ensure an acceptable level, there should be a proper balance between factors which raise blood glucose and those which lower it. Blood glucose rises after a meal, and blood glucose falls as a result of fasting, exercise, insulin or OHA. Therefore any change in routine which is likely to lower blood glucose should be compensated by taking food before it is too late. If some delay has already occurred in taking corrective action, then the food should be such that it will raise blood glucose rapidly: such a 'food' is four teaspoons of glucose or sugar.

Hypoglycemia may be prevented by taking the following precautions:

1. No meal should be missed, or made much lighter than the one on which good blood glucose control has been achieved.
2. If one is expecting unusual physical effort, it should be compensated by taking extra food before the effort. As a

precaution against unexpected effort, some food (such as biscuits) or sugar should be carried all the time.
3. If one is expecting unusual physical effort, missing a dose of insulin or OHA may not help because most drugs have a duration of action of 12-24 hours, and therefore the previous dose taken about 12 hours earlier might produce the hypoglycemia.
4. If one is expecting that a meal will have to be missed (eg when one has to go for a fasting blood test), at least one dose of the drug should be missed. For example, if one has to go fasting for a medical test in the morning, that morning's dose of insulin/OHA should not be taken.
5. If at bedtime, self-monitoring of blood glucose reveals a value less than 110 mg/dL, a bedtime snack should be taken to prevent hypoglycemia during the middle of the night. Hypoglycemia during sleep is particularly dangerous since many of the early symptoms may be missed.

Treatment

If the early symptoms of hypoglycemia are noticed, the condition may be easily treated by taking four teaspoons of glucose or sugar dissolved in a small quantity of water. If neither glucose nor sugar is available, eating some candy, jam, biscuits, honey, bread or rice is also much better than having nothing.

If early symptoms have been missed, one should give the patient one of the above things to eat, and in the meantime seek medical help.

If the detection of hypoglycemia has been delayed so much that the patient is on the verge of losing consciousness, or has actually lost it, giving anything through the mouth is first difficult (because the patient cannot swallow), and secondly dangerous (because anything put into the mouth may go to the lungs and interfere with breathing). In such a situation, 25g of glucose is given by intravenous injection in the form of a 50% solution (i.e. 25g glucose dissolved in 50 ml sterile water). Since intravenous (i.v.) injections need much more skill than intramuscular (i.m.) or subcutaneous (s.c.) injections, in an emergency another alternative is to give glucagon (1 mg) by i.m. or s.c. injection. (Glucagon has no similarity with glucose. Glucagon is a hormone which has actions quite opposite those of insulin).

Experience does not necessarily help

Those having diabetes generally learn to recognise the early symptoms of hypoglycemia and can take timely corrective action. But two factors might make it difficult even for highly experienced diabetics to detect hypoglycemia in time:
   (a) Long-standing diabetes is often associated with autonomic neuropathy because of which early warning symptoms such as palpitation and sweating may be weak or absent.
   (b) If the person is taking beta-blockers for hypertension, the drugs weaken the early warning symptoms.

Skin and foot care

In diabetes, infections often get prolonged. Further, because of peripheral neuropathy, injuries fail to cause much pain, and may therefore escape attention. Hence the best one can do is to prevent injuries and infection, for which the following precautions are useful:
1. Have a bath everyday.
2. Keep the skin dry, specially the folds, such as the axillae, groin, the space between fingers and between toes. After bathing, dry these parts carefully and dust them with talcum powder.
3. Be careful to avoid injuries during shaving or paring nails.
4. Do not cut the nails too short, specially at the ends.
5. Treat any injury or skin infection promptly.
6. Do not use socks with very tight elastic bands.
7. Wear well-fitting shoes. The shoes should be a little loose.
8. When sitting cross-legged, shift the leg frequently.
9. While lying down, spend some time with the feet raised with the help of a support.

10. Keep the teeth clean by brushing twice a day, and rinsing the mouth with water after eating anything.
11. Contact the doctor if there is numbness or tingling in the limbs, pain in the calves while walking, or change in the colour of nails, toes or the skin anywhere else.

Regular check-up

The treatment of diabetes with insulin and OHA has made it possible for a diabetic to have a normal life span. But these agents to not restore complete normalcy, thereby making a diabetic prone to several serious complications. Therefore living a productive long life needs eternal vigilance. The need for regular check-ups is further increased by the fact that complications such as hypertension and retinopathy are silent to start with, and neuropathy makes the detection of complications such as angina difficult by taking away the capacity for feeling pain. Besides maintaining a daily diary (see below) and daily self-monitoring of blood glucose (see below), the patient should visit his doctor regularly as indicated in Table 3. Besides these regular check-ups, additional visits may be required as and when there is a specific complaint such as a skin infection, deterioration of vision, or deterioration in the control of blood glucose.

TABLE 3. CHECK-UPS DESIRABLE IN DIABETES

Check-up	Frequency
Body weight	Every 3 months
Blood glucose	Every 3 months
Glycated haemoglobin	Every 3 months
Examination of legs and feet	Every 6 months
Blood cholesterol	Once a year
Urine for macro- and micro-albuminuria	Once a year
Eye examination (including fundus examination)	Once a year

It is also desirable to attend an authentic patient education programme once a year to revise what one may already know, and to learn new things.

Stress management

Stress releases hormones which have actions somewhat opposite to those of insulin. Therefore stress increases the risk of diabetes. And, if diabetes is already present, stress can make it worse. There are many techniques and prescriptions available for overcoming stress, but the most handy and potent is positive thinking. Positive thinking depends on the inner resources of the individual, and is therefore always available. The situation may not change, but the person feels better because he starts looking at it differently. The freedom to look at things the way we like is always available to us. Using this strategy we can always refuse to be miserable. Even when we cannot stretch logic to the point of looking at a thoroughly hopeless situation positively, spiritual disciplines such as yoga enable us to view the situation positively.

Diabetic diary and card

Every diabetic patient should maintain a diary. The first page should have his name, date of birth, address, phone, blood group, information about allergies (if any), his doctor/hospital's name, address, phone, etc., and an alternative address and phone on which somebody may be contacted in case of an emergency. The next few pages should have the latest insulin/OHA routine being followed. Every time the treatment is revised, it should be recorded along with the date on which the change was made. The next few pages should have in a tabular form the readings of regular check-ups such as body weight, blood pressure, urine examination, and blood examination along with the date of the test. The rest of the diary should have in a tabular form the blood glucose level along with the date and time at which it was done.

The diabetic should always carry a card in his pocket/purse. The card should have the same information as on the first page of the diary. In addition, it should have an appeal requesting that if the person is found drowsy or behaving abnormally, he may be given sugar or something sweet, and if the person is found unconscious, he should be taken to a doctor or a hospital. Some sugar or candy should preferably be kept in the patient's purse or pocket all the time.

YOGA AND DIABETES

Yoga is an enlightened way of life based on a spiritual view of life. It has all the elements of a healthy lifestyle discussed above, besides much more. To elaborate, it includes regular exercise, a prudent diet, and stress reduction. In addition, a person following a yogic lifestyle is unlikely to smoke or drink because for him the reasons for which people generally smoke or drink cease to exist. Further, when a person follows a disciplined and sensible lifestyle based on yoga, he enjoys it rather than feel deprived of the pleasures of life. Thus yoga has tremendous potential for the prevention and treatment of diabetes. However, it would be incorrect to look at yoga as an alternative to insulin or OHA. Depending on the severity or the type of diabetes, insulin or OHA may or may not be required along with yoga. If medication is still necessary, yoga is likely to reduce the dose of insulin or OHA required, and moreover, yoga can bring a positive outlook towards life, diabetes notwithstanding.

CONCLUSION

Managing diabetes is essentially a balancing act – balancing factors which raise blood glucose with those which lower it so that the net result is blood glucose level in the normal range (Fig. 11.3). However, how these factors are balanced is also important. To eat carelessly, not exercise and to live in perpetual worry, anxiety and fear, and then to achieve a balance by taking a high dose of insulin or OHA does not give the best results. Food should be just

FACTORS WHICH RAISE BLOOD GLUCOSE

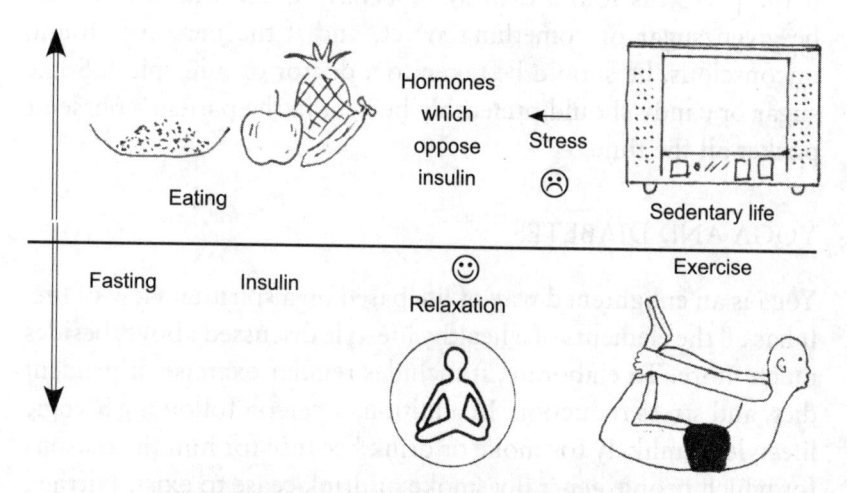

Eating — Hormones which oppose insulin ← Stress — Sedentary life

Fasting — Insulin — Relaxation — Exercise

FACTORS WHICH LOWER BLOOD GLUCOSE

Fig. 11.3. *Normal blood glucose is the result of a balance between factors which raise blood glucose and those which lower it. Knowledge of these factors is particularly important for a person having diabetes.*

adequate in quantity, not excessive. The quality of food should be such that the rise in blood glucose following each meal is modest. On the other side of the balance, moderate exercise is essential so that there is no undue dependence on insulin or OHA to keep the blood glucose in check.

Frequently Asked Questions

1. *How important is it to pay attention to the diet if insulin or tablets are used for diabetes?*

    It is very important. Insulin or OHA tables are not a substitute for a prudent diet. To try and compensate for a careless diet by taking an extra dose of the drug is inviting fate, and fate can be very cruel in the case of diabetes.

2. *Can a diabetic observe a fast?*

    Yes, if he is not on medication. In fact, if he is overweight, and not on medication, regular fasting would do him good. But if a diabetic on medication observes a fast, his blood glucose may fall to a dangerously low level. Therefore one alternative is that he should not fast. The second alternative is to miss two doses of the drug: one which he normally takes half an hour before the meal he plans to miss during the fast, *and also* the dose which he takes 6-12 hours before that. For example, if he plans to miss breakfast, he should miss the morning dose *as well as* the previous night's dose.

3. *Which are the foods a diabetic should avoid?*

    The traditional list of such foods is very long, and includes sugar, rice, potatoes, bananas, mango, chickoo, grapes, etc. But there is no scientific basis for any of these foods to be strictly forbidden. Sugar has already been discussed in detail. The following principles which apply to sugar intake also hold for all the other notorious foods, viz:
    a. have it in moderation;
    b. take it as part of a meal, not alone; and
    c. take into account the calories it gives while calculating the day's intake

4. *Can a diabetic have tea and coffee?*

    He does not have to, but can have these in moderation if he wants to. If he sweetens them with sugar, greater restraint is required in order to limit the sugar intake. In any case, the caloric content of the milk and sugar in the tea/coffee should be taken into account while calculating the daily energy intake.

5. *Is fructose better than sugar for diabetics?*

    Fructose is the sugar in fruits. The general population as well as diabetics can take fruits without any hesitation. However, foods to which fructose has been added instead of ordinary sugar are not necessarily better for diabetics. In the long run, fructose can raise blood levels of triglycerides and LDL cholesterol. Further, large amounts of fructose may cause an upset stomach.

6. *Are low calorie sweeteners safe for diabetics?*

As the name indicates, low calorie sweeteners are sweet like sugar but do not provide much energy. Two types of compounds satisfy these requirements: bulk sweeteners and high intensity sweeteners. Bulk sweeteners cannot contribute to energy supply because they are indigestible. High intensity sweeteners are so sweet that just a few milligrams may sweeten a food as much as a spoonful of sugar. Since bulk sweeteners may be fermented in the intestines, they may cause flatulence. In that sense, high intensity sweeteners are better. Saccharin, a long-known high intensity sweetener has always been shrouded in controversy. The most popular today is aspartame, and is in all likelihood completely safe. However, now that diabetics are allowed a moderate amount of sugar, the significance of sweeteners has gone down. However, sweeteners have another advantage: their calorific value is negligible. Whether it is desirable to try to get the sweet taste somehow instead of developing self-control is an issue every individual has to decide for himself.

7. *What are diabetic foods?*

The term 'diabetic foods' is misleading. Neither can these foods be eaten by a diabetic in unrestricted amounts, nor do they contribute to the treatment of diabetes. They are merely sweetened foods which contain a low calorie sweetener instead of sugar. But their constituents other than the sweetener do provide energy, and these should be taken into account. With these qualifications, diabetic foods may be harmless, but they are not particularly worth recommending.

8. *Is acarbose good for diabetes?*

   Acarbose inhibits carbohydrate digestion. As a result, if a person takes acarbose, the starch in his food will not be completely digested. The incompletely digested starch is not absorbed, and therefore does not raise blood sugar. Thus one can eat, and yet avoid the rise in blood sugar. This sounds very attractive but two important points to consider are as follows:
   a. The incompletely digested starch reaches the large intestine where it is utilised by bacteria. In the process, gases are released. Therefore acarbose produces flatulence.
   b. The purpose of eating is to digest and absorb food in order to nourish the body, not to enjoy it while it is in the mouth. What one is trying to accomplish with acarbose can be simply accomplished by eating less.

9. *Are there some specific asanas which cure diabetes?*

   There are no asanas that can cure diabetes. But in mild cases of diabetes, asanas, like other physical activities, may restore normal blood glucose levels if coupled with diet control and weight loss. Regarding the specificity of asanas, a few which involve turning and twisting of the abdomen such as *ardhamatsyendrasana, bhujangasana* and *dhanurasana* are recommended. But it is worthwhile to remember that a diabetic is more a person than diabetes. He also needs a healthy heart, liver, intestines and spine as much as anybody else. Therefore it is much better to establish a routine involving a judicious selection of 15-20 asanas instead of focusing on a few 'meant for diabetes'. Why not use diabetes as an excuse for getting healthy generally!

10. *What is the blood glucose level a diabetic should aim at?*

    A diabetic should balance his diet, drugs and physical activity in such a way as to maintain fasting blood glucose at about

130 mg/dL and peak postprandial blood glucose below 180 mg/dL. These values are close to the upper limit of what is normal. A diabetic need not aim at values lower than this:
a. to avoid hypoglycemia, and
b. because the brain of a diabetic gets used to high blood glucose. Hence lower values, which may otherwise be within the normal range, might produce in these persons symptoms of hypoglycemia.

11. *What is the relationship between urine glucose and blood glucose?*

The fasting blood glucose is normally about 100 mg/dL, and after meals the peak blood glucose is about 150 mg/dL. So as long as the blood glucose stays below 180 mg/dL, it does not appear in the urine. Therefore the absence of glucose in the urine is no guarantee that everything is normal. But the presence of glucose in the urine means that blood glucose is abnormally high – in order to know exactly how high, an estimation of blood glucose is necessary. Although urine glucose has very limited value, it is often done because it is so much more convenient to check than blood glucose.

12. *What is ketosis?*

In diabetes, the ability to utilise carbohydrates is impaired. Therefore the body starts using fats to get energy. Using too much fat and too little carbohydrate for energy produces an abundance of chemicals called ketones, and the condition is called ketosis. Ketosis is a sign of severe uncontrolled diabetes. Ketones impart a characteristic smell to the urine and can be detected by a chemical test on the urine. The presence of ketones in the urine is a warning for urgent action, failing which the person might lapse into unconsciousness. This unconsciousness is associated with a very high blood glucose level (hyperglycemia), and therefore cannot be corrected by giving glucose. Instead it needs insulin for treatment, and is best treated by a doctor rather than the patient himself. However, when in doubt whether unconsciousness is due to hypoglycemia or due to hyperglycemia, it is much safer to give glucose than insulin.

13. *What is the role of heredity in diabetes?*

    The role is substantial: anybody whose parents have diabetes has a 50 per cent chance of getting diabetes, and if only one of the parents has diabetes, the child has a 25 per cent chance of getting diabetes. However, heredity produces only a tendency towards getting diabetes, not the disease itself. Exactly at what age the disease will manifest, and how severe it will be, depends to a large extent on the lifestyle of the person. With a proper lifestyle, a person with a strong inherited tendency towards diabetes may be able to avoid the disease altogether, delay its onset, or at least reduce its severity. Finally, it does not help to worry; worry only increases the chances of getting the disease. The constructive approach to the situation is to do what one can, and not to worry about what one cannot help.

14. *Can some plant products or indigenous drugs cure diabetes?*

    There are hundreds of edible plants, medicinal plants and indigenous drugs which might be of some use in diabetes. But those trained in modern scientific medicine know very little about such treatments. However, the following general comments are pertinent:
    a. If a curative drug existed, it would have been widely known.
    b. Many patients who have tried these products have been disappointed. Apparently, these products are overrated by those who prescribe them.
    c. There is a popular feeling that plant products and indigenous drugs at least do no harm. This assumption is not entirely valid. No drug is completely safe.

d. The pharmacology and dosage of indigenous drugs are not as well worked out as those of modern drugs.
e. The limited studies that have been done indicate that:
   (i) the potency of indigenous drugs or beneficial plants is weaker than that of insulin or OHA, and therefore may help only cases of mild diabetes,
   (ii) overdose of indigenous drugs may also produce hypoglycemia like insulin or OHA,
   (iii) indigenous drugs also have to be taken lifelong, and are in that sense not curative, and
   (iv) indigenous drugs are not necessarily less expensive than insulin or OHA.
f. The possibility of at least some indigenous drugs having special merit exists. Recent research done by the Indian Council of Medical Research (ICMR) has given encouraging results with *methi* (fenugreek), *jamun* (Eugenia jambolana) and *vijaysar* (Pterocarpus marsupium). More research is needed on these and other promising substances such as *karela* (bitter gourd), *neem*, *bael*, etc.

15. *What is gestational diabetes?*

Gestational diabetes is diabetes during pregnancy. The metabolic changes of pregnancy are conducive to produce diabetes. Therefore diabetes may be detected in a woman for the first time during pregnancy. If left untreated, diabetes of the mother can harm the baby. Therefore every pregnant woman should get an oral glucose tolerance test (OGTT) done every 3 months during pregnancy. Many of the women who get gestational diabetes become 'normal' after pregnancy. But any woman who gets gestational diabetes has a greater than 50% chance of developing diabetes later in life. Gestational diabetes should therefore be taken as a warning bell for improving the lifestyle, and losing some weight, if necessary. On the other hand, if a woman with established diabetes gets pregnant, the diabetes is likely to get worse during pregnancy.

This is bad for both the mother and the baby. Therefore close monitoring is essential in such cases. However, with proper care, a diabetic woman can go through the pregnancy normally, and deliver a normal baby.

16. *Are there any special precautions a diabetic should observe during an illness such as fever?*

    Illness is a stress, and in all stressful situations, diabetes tends to get worse. Therefore if a diabetic is on insulin or OHA, these should not be stopped during an illness. At the same time, food should not be stopped. If solid foods are difficult to take, one may shift to semi-solids and liquids. But continuing with insulin or OHA in the absence of adequate food intake poses the risk of hypoglycemia.
    On the other hand, if no change is made in medication and diet, worsening of diabetes in illness might lead to hyperglycemia, and even ketosis. If the urine shows the presence of ketones, medical advice should be urgently sought.

Suggested Reading

Raghuram TC, Pasricha S, Sharma RD, *Diet and Diabetes*. Hyderabad: National Institute of Nutrition, 1991. (Available at ICMR, New Delhi).

12

Breathe Easy

Life is not a laughing matter – but can you imagine having to live without laughing.

LEONID SUKHORUKOV

Breathing is a sign of life, and the essence of life. No wonder, difficulty in breathing makes us uneasy and may be viewed with a good deal of anxiety and fear. A recurring difficulty in breathing, as in bronchial asthma, therefore leads to considerable mental stress. Paradoxically, the stress itself may make the asthma worse. On the other hand, hope and happiness can make the life of an asthmatic much easier. Understanding the disease, avoiding the triggers for an attack, and listening to the body for warning signals enable a person having asthma to lead an essentially normal, highly productive and enjoyable life with less medication.

OUR RESPIRATORY SYSTEM

Our body is like an engine. It treats much of our food as fuel and burns (oxidises) it to obtain energy. Oxygen is essential for the oxidation of food, and carbon dioxide is produced as a waste product during the process. The respiratory system carries fresh oxygen to the body, and removes carbon dioxide from the body.

The air has about 20 per cent oxygen. When the air reaches our lungs, a part of this oxygen is transferred to the blood, which in turn carries it to different parts of the body. The same blood in the lungs has the carbon dioxide which it has brought from different parts of the body. A part of this carbon dioxide is transferred to the lungs and thrown out when we breathe out. That is why the air that we breathe out has less than 20 per cent oxygen and has a considerable quantity of carbon dioxide (Fig. 12.1).

■ Oxygen   ■ Nitrogen   ■ Carbondioxide

INSPIRED AIR   EXPIRED AIR

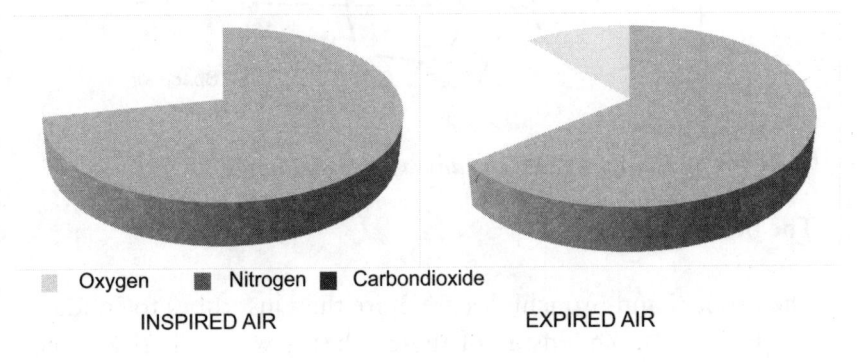

Fig. 12.1. *The composition of inspired and expired air.*

A crucial step in the process of respiration, therefore, is to carry the air to the lungs and to take it out after the gaseous exchange. The job of conducting the air in and out of the lungs is done by the airways. The airways begin with the nose and continue into a rather wide windpipe (trachea). The trachea can be felt in front of the neck. The trachea divides into two bronchi, which in turn divide into smaller tubes called bronchioles (Fig. 12.2). The process of repeated division continues, much like the branches of a tree. It is the exaggerated sensitivity of these branches which is the hallmark of bronchial asthma.

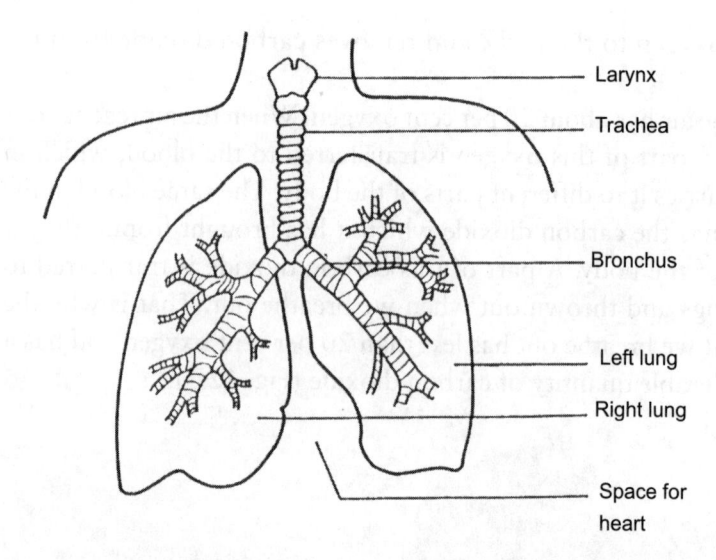

Fig. 12.2. *The airway tree and lungs.*

The bronchial tree

The bronchi and bronchioles are more than just tubes to conduct air (Fig. 12.3). The inside of these tubes is wet and sticky, and has fine hair (called cilia). Dust particles entering the airways stick to the wet and sticky surface, and are swept upwards by the cilia. Thus only clean air reaches the lungs. Germs entering the airways are often trapped and killed in the airways by cells specially equipped to do so. Thus germs generally do not reach the lungs. Particles larger than dust, and a variety of chemicals, irritate the airways. The irritation leads to contraction of the muscle in the walls of the airways. That in turn brings about narrowing of the airways. Narrowing of the airways prevents particles from reaching the lungs. Irritation of the airways also increases the formation of the sticky liquid (mucus) in their walls. As a result, the particle may be dissolved, or the irritant chemical gets diluted. Thus the constriction of the airways and the secretion of mucus are protective mechanisms primarily designed to defend the lungs.

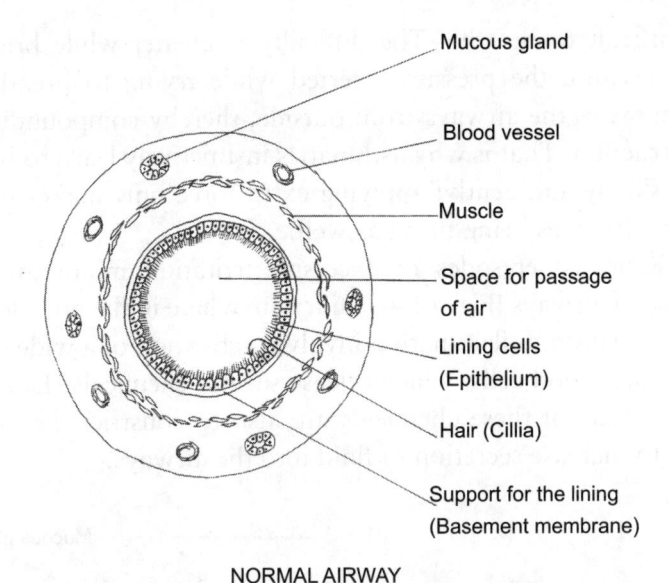

Fig. 12.3. *A diagrammatic sketch of the structure of a normal airway. This is how its cut surface looks under a microscope if the airway is cut across.*

SMOKING DOES NOT LET THE LUNGS WORK

Among the various ill effects of smoking is the paralysing effect it has on airway defence mechanisms. Smoking paralyses the cilia and injures the cells which engulf germs and foreign particles. Further, smoking irritates the airways, thereby constricting the airways and filling them with extra fluid. These effects are harmful for all; for a person having asthma, they are a disaster.

WHAT HAPPENS IN BRONCHIAL ASTHMA

In the case of bronchial asthma, the airways are highly sensitive. As a result, some of the mechanisms primarily designed to defend the lungs become harmful; excess of even a good thing can be bad. A wide variety of stimuli may bring about a strong constriction of the airways and a massive increase in formation of the sticky liquid (mucus). Both these effects block the airways, making it difficult to breathe. The difficulty is greater while breathing out because the pressure exerted while trying to breathe out compresses the airways from outside, thereby compounding the obstruction. That is why asthmatics instinctively learn to breathe out slowly and gently: applying extra force only makes matters worse (besides being tiring as well).

Repeated episodes of excessive irritation injure the inner lining of airways (Fig. 12.4). Injury anywhere in the body leads to inflammation. Inflammation involves activation of a wide variety of white blood cells, which release several chemicals (Fig. 12.5). The effects of these chemicals are also to constrict the airways and to increase secretion of fluid into the airways.

AIRWAY IN BRONCHIAL ASTHMA

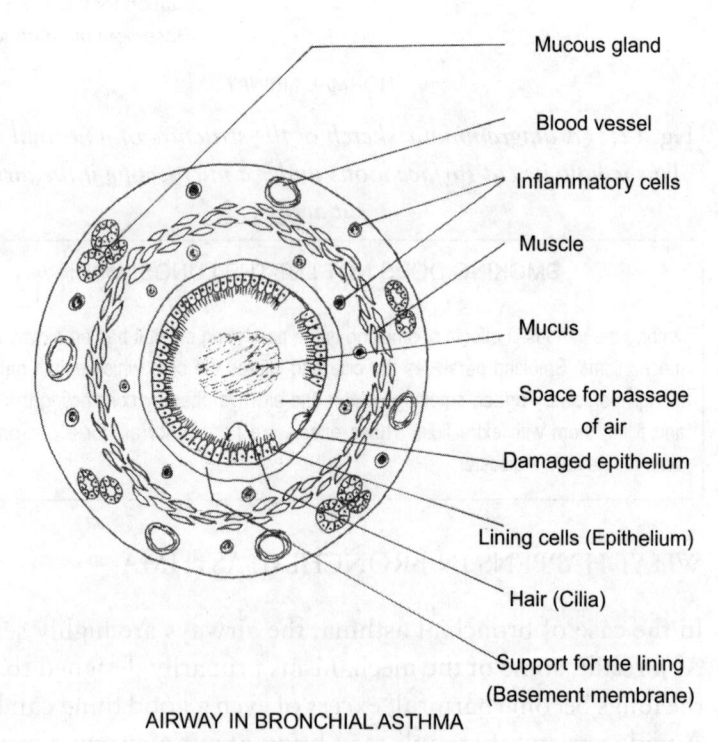

Fig. 12.4. *A diagrammatic sketch of the structure of an airway in bronchial asthma. This is how its cut surface looks under a microscope if the airway is cut across.*

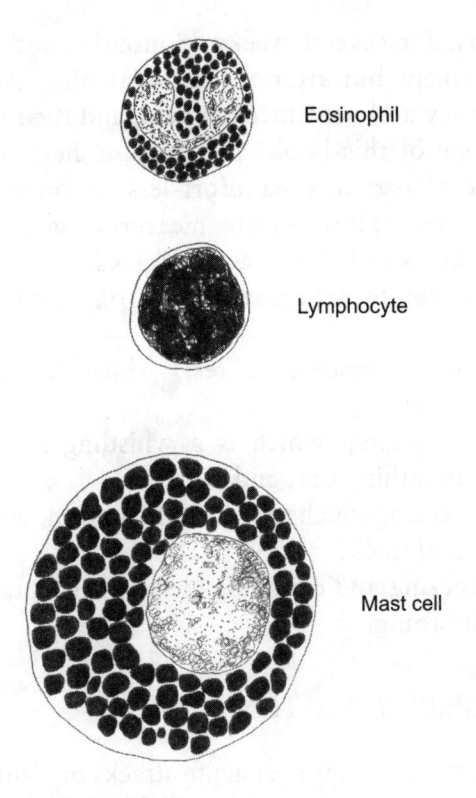

Fig. 12.5. Cells *activated in bronchial asthma. Eosinophils and lymphocytes are types of white blood cells. Mast cells are close cousins of white blood cells found in airways and many other parts of the body. These three cell types are the principal culprits which, on activation, release chemicals which bring on the symptoms of bronchial asthma.*

Symptoms

Although there are various types and varying grades of asthma, it is generally a chronic disease with alternating phases of symptomatic and relatively normal periods. The symptomatic periods are further of two types: *acute attacks* which have to be treated as an emergency, and which can generally be controlled within a few hours; and *chronic phases* of discomfort which may last for several weeks or months, and make everyday life inconvenient but are not life-threatening. Acute attacks are an emergency and need medical help, and their treatment is beyond the scope of this book. The purpose here is to help you make chronic phases of discomfort less uncomfortable, shorter, and less frequent. However, the measures suggested here would also reduce the possibility of acute attacks.

The symptomatic phases of chronic asthma are characterised by:
  (a) breathlessness at rest, which increases with physical exertion,
  (b) wheezing, which is a whistling sound produced while breathing out, and
  (c) cough, which may include sputum, which is usually white and thick.

Wheezing and coughing are at their worst at night and early in the morning.

TRIGGERS FOR ASTHMA

The factors which trigger acute attacks of asthma or make chronic phases worse may be uncontrollable or unavoidable, but are not entirely unpredictable. Recognising them, and avoiding them to the extent possible is an important part of treatment. The most frequent triggers have been listed below:

1. Allergens

The common allergens are pollen grains, dust mites, fur, feathers, animal danders, and moulds (fungi).

2. Irritants

The common irritants are cold air, dust, tobacco smoke (even someone else smoking nearby can be a nuisance), industrial pollutants and vehicular pollutants.

3. Infections

Respiratory infections, specially viral infections, are frequent triggers for asthma.

4. Exercise

The likelihood of exercise triggering an asthmatic attack increases with its intensity. Thus running is more likely to trigger an attack than walking. Further, inhaling cold and dry air during exercise makes matters worse.

5. Occupational hazards

If one's occupation involves exposure to chemicals or dusts, they could be among the triggers for precipitating asthma.

6. Drugs

Beta blockers, commonly used for heart disease and high blood pressure, constrict bronchi. Therefore they are not given if a person also has asthma. In addition, aspirin and other similar drugs used for relieving pain, inflammation or fever, may also trigger an asthmatic attack.

7. Emotional stress

Emotional stress makes asthma worse. Conversely, positive emotions improve asthma. Besides the clinical association between emotions and asthma, which has been known for a long time, now there are also plausible biological mechanisms known which may be responsible for the association.

TREATMENT OF BRONCHIAL ASTHMA

Asthma can be treated successfully and the life of the patient can be quite comfortable if the disease is treated with respect and understanding, and not fear. The treatment involves several aspects, all of them important in their own way.

1. Drug treatment

Asthma involves two basic pathologic processes: the narrowing of airways (bronchoconstriction), and the inflammation of the airways. Accordingly, two types of drugs are commonly used in asthma: those which relax bronchial muscles and thereby widen the airways (bronchodilators), and those which reduce inflammation (anti-inflammatory drugs). Fortunately, very effective drugs are now available in both categories. Drugs of either category can be administered by three routes in asthma: by inhalation, orally, or by injection.

Inhalation is the best route of administration. The effect is immediate because the drug is delivered exactly where it is required. For the same reason, the dose required is the smallest, and therefore side effects (such as tremors) are minimal. Hence doctors prefer inhalers for treating asthma. But some patients associate an inhaler with a serious, life-threatening situation. But at least in the case of asthma, this is not true. An inhaler may be required even for the mildest form of the disease in the case of asthma, and may be the only treatment required for many patients.

Patients love pills, but in case of asthma doctors prescribe them only if inhalers are not enough. Injections are reserved for emergencies, and should be administered only under medical supervision. Different forms of drug treatment have been compared in Table 1.

Since the severity of the disease changes with time, season, and the presence of various triggering factors, periodic check ups are required for the revision of drug treatment. Besides what the patient reports, doctors frequently depend on two breathing tests to determine whether tablets are required in addition to inhalers, how many, and in what dose. One of the tests measures the maximum rate of air flow while breathing out forcefully (Peak Expiratory Flow Rate, or PEFR). The other test measures the volume of air breathed out during the first second of a forceful expiration (Forced Expiratory Volume in one second, or FEV_1).

TABLE 1. A COMPARISON OF DIFFERENT ROUTES OF DRUG DELIVERY IN CASE OF BRONCHIAL ASTHMA

	Inhalers	Tablets	Injections
Rapidity of action	Immediate	Delayed	Immediate
Duration of action	Short/long	Long	Long
Side effects	Less	More	More
Convenient	Yes	Yes	No
Indication	Mild attack	Given in moderate and severe cases along with inhalers	Emergency, i.e. a severe attack
Frequency	As and when required	Fixed dose 2-3 times a day, as prescribed by the doctor	As and when required

2. Avoiding likely triggers

The first trigger to avoid is cigarette smoke. An asthmatic who continues to smoke has only himself to blame for his misery. There are no drugs which can make an asthmatic smoker comfortable.

The other triggers which can be avoided with some success are cold air, fur, feathers, undue exertion, drugs and emotional stress. To avoid pollen grains, one should avoid exposure to flowering vegetation, and keep windows closed during extreme weather. To avoid dust mites, one should wash bedding with hot water regularly. The bedroom should be well ventilated, and sun allowed in for at least some time everyday. Carpets should be avoided, specially in the bedroom, since dust tends to collect under them. Also, avoid keeping pets in the house. If there are some items in the diet which show a clear association with asthmatic attacks, those items should be given up. If the asthma is clearly related to exposure to some chemicals in the course of one's work, a serious thought should be given to change of occupation.

3. Hyposensitisation

If a specific allergen is clearly known (eg a pollen grain or a chemical), which is usually *not* the case, a procedure called hyposensitisation is sometimes helpful. In this procedure a very small quantity of the allergen is injected. After a few days, a slightly larger quantity is injected. In this way several injections of gradually increasing dose of the allergen are given at regular interval. By this process, the person gradually gets 'accustomed' to the allergen, and does not react to it as violently as he did previously. The procedure carries a small risk of precipitating an allergic response soon after the injection. Besides this, its efficacy is limited. Moreover, most patients are allergic to a large number of allergens, and it is not practical to hyposensitise the patient to all of them. Finally, to discover all the allergens to which a patient is sensitive is almost impossible. Because of all these reasons, hyposensitisation is not a very popular procedure and is not routinely recommended in cases of asthma.

4. Yoga

Yoga is a comprehensive change of attitude and lifestyle. Several aspects of yoga may be logically expected to help bronchial asthma as explained below:

(a) *Yogasanas* and *pranayama* involve breathing discipline which is likely to improve respiratory function.

(b) Yoga involves giving up smoking. Further, it also provides a solution to the mental stress which may result from giving up smoking.

(c) If the treatment requires giving up certain specific foods, the yogic attitude makes it easy to do so without suffering mental stress in the process.

(d) Yoga is likely to help other diseases, thereby reducing the need for beta blockers or pain killers, which may trigger asthma.

(e) Yoga is likely to improve one's immune status, which would reduce the frequency of respiratory infections which may trigger an asthma attack.

(f) Last but not least, yoga enables us to view life differently. As a result, many things simply cease to matter, thereby leading to stress reduction, and positive feelings. The improvement in emotional health can bring about a remarkable reduction in the severity of asthma and the frequency of attacks.

Although not much research has been done on the subject, the few studies that are available are all consistent in finding that yoga does actually help patients having bronchial asthma significantly.

CLOSING THOUGHTS

An individual, with all parts the body perfect, does not exist. But in spite of that, we survive, and often quite well. What really matters is that we should be able to go about our routine with ease, be without pain or discomfort, and feel happy. Some physical handicap may make it difficult for us to do certain things, but what is important is that there are still many things that we can do very well, and that is enough. Everyone cannot do everything, and *need not* do everything. For example, everyone need not be a mountain climber or a good singer. The world runs largely with the help of very ordinary people. We should first realise our strengths and weaknesses and then should organise our life in such a way that we can make the best use of our strengths. If we are able to do that, we can create a niche for ourselves, and that is a major determinant of happiness. If we are happy, our physical handicaps cease to matter.

Frequently Asked Questions

1. *Is asthma curable?*

   It is not, but that is not as terrible as it looks. We all have some weak points in the body which trouble us. But that need not necessarily make us miserable. Enjoy the present. Don't let past discomfort or possibility of future pain spoil the present. That way, life itself is an incurable disease: its only cure is death, and we are all interested in postponing the cure as much as possible!

2. *Can herbs cure asthma?*

   Those trained in modern scientific medicine do not know much about herbs. However, the following general observations are pertinent:
   (a) If a curative herb was there, it would have been widely known.
   (b) Many patients who have used certain herbs in the hope of getting cured have been disappointed. Apparently, herbs are overrated by those who prescribe them.
   (c) There is a popular feeling that at least herbs can do no

harm. This assumption is not entirely valid. Herbs, like drugs, are chemicals, and can have side effects.

(d) The pharmacology and dosage of herbs is often not as standardised as that of modern drugs.

(e) Herbal treatments, like any other treatment, could have at least some of their efficacy because of making the patient feel that something helpful has been done ('psychological'/ 'placebo' effect).

(f) The possibility of at least some herbs helping some patients exists. It is an avenue open for much fruitful research.

13

The Poor Back

> *Pain is the hand of Nature sculpturing men to greatness: an inspired labour chisels with heavenly cruelty an unwilling mould.*
>
> SRI AUROBINDO

More than 80 per cent of us experience back pain at least once in life. However, it is neither inevitable nor incurable. Back pain is largely preventable, and even if prevention fails, it can be generally treated successfully without undergoing a surgery.

PHYSICAL BASIS OF BACK PAIN

It is often said that back pain is the price human beings have to pay for an erect posture. It is believed that the erect posture imposes a load on the lower back that is too heavy for it to bear. But that is not strictly true. First, as we go down the spine, the diameter of the vertebrae increases, thereby making it stable and capable of withstanding heavy loads: this is a structural adaptation unique to human beings and their erect posture (Fig. 13.1). Secondly, the spine is well supported by muscles and ligaments so that it can combine flexibility and mobility with strength and stability. In

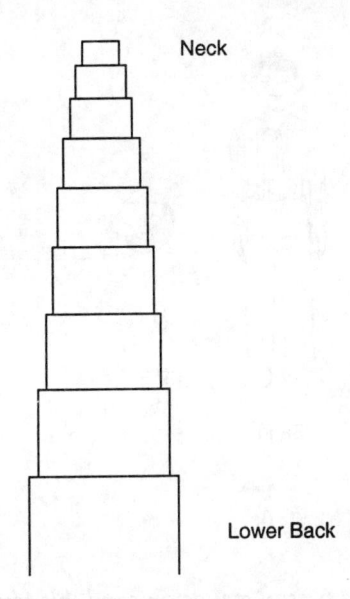

Fig. 13.1. *The vertebrae get wider as we go down the back.*

order to understand the role of muscles, going into a bit of physics is essential. What the structure of the back has to withstand is not actually the load, but the pressure generated by the load. The pressure is the load acting on unit area of the surface. If the area on which the load is imposed increases, the pressure becomes less. The implications of this fact may be illustrated by an example. If a person stands in a sand pit, his feet sink. If the same person lies down in the same pit, he hardly makes any dent on the surface of the sand (Fig. 13.2). Although the weight of the person remains the same, its impact is much greater when the weight acts on a small surface (feet). That is because pressure is equal to the force divided by the area.

Now let us come back to the back. When we lift a load, the muscles of the back and abdomen reflexly undergo contraction: you can feel the tightening of the tummy and flanks while lifting the load. The result is that the back along with these muscles (and the ribs) convert the body into a hard cylinder. The weight of the

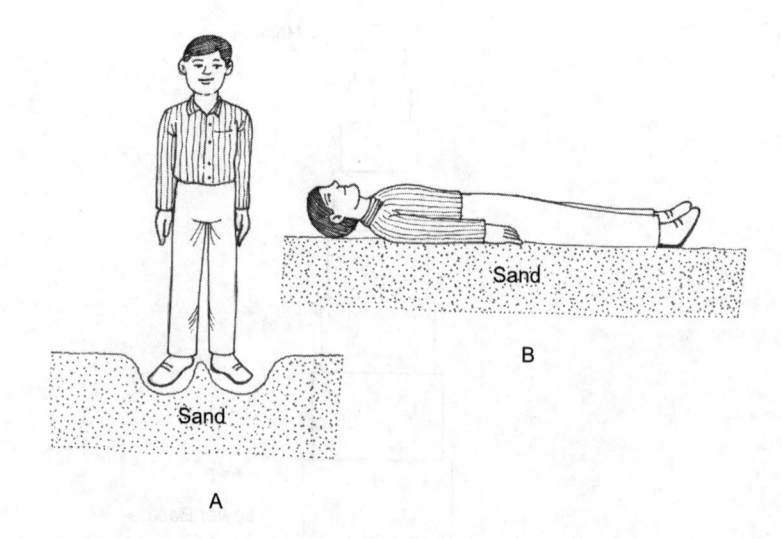

Fig. 13.2. *If a person stands on sand, his feet sink into it, making deep depressions in the sand (A). If he lies down on the sand (B), there is hardly any effect on the surface of the sand.*

load is imposed on the whole cylinder, not just on the backbone. Thus the pressure on the bony structures is reduced (Fig. 13.3). That is the reason why back pain is more likely if the muscles of the back and abdomen are weak; conversely, strengthening these muscles through appropriate exercises is a part of the treatment of backache. That is also the reason why back injuries are most likely if a load lands suddenly on the back so that there is no time for the abdominal and back muscles to contract. This can happen when we slip while walking, or if we suddenly support someone near us if he or she falls.

THE STRUCTURE OF THE BACK

The structure of the back is admirably suited to the three functions it has to perform. First, it has to be strong because it bears the weight of the body as well as the weight of the load we carry.

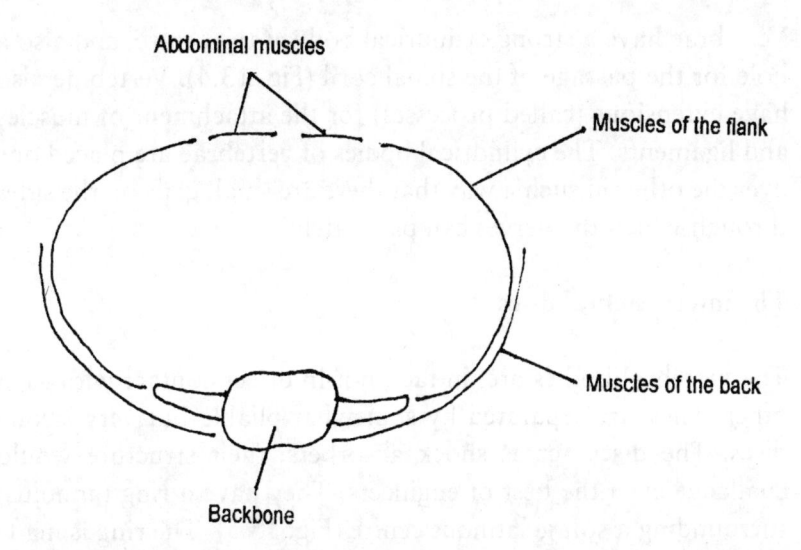

Fig. 13.3. *When we carry a load, the weight is distributed throughout the cylinder made up by the backbone, muscles of the back and flank, and abdominal muscles. Lifting the load leads to reflex contraction of these muscles, thereby making the cylinder hard.*

Secondly, it has to be flexible so that the back can bend forwards, backwards and sideways, and also twist around its axis. Finally, the backbone has to accommodate the spinal cord, allow passage to the nerves issuing from the spinal cord, and protect these neural structures. The spinal cord is an extension of the brain, is a delicate structure, and is also an important structure since an injury to it may lead to paralysis. The needs of a strong structure are somewhat contradictory to those of a structure which is flexible and protective. The back is so made that it is able to perform all these functions admirably well for a whole lifetime. In most people, for most of the time, the back does not fail.

The vertebral column

The back has in the midline, the backbone (vertebral column) which is made up of a series of ring-like bones (vertebrae).

Vertebrae have a strong cylindrical body at the centre, and also a hole for the passage of the spinal cord (Fig. 13.4). Vertebrae also have extensions (called processes) for the attachment of muscles and ligaments. The cylindrical bodies of vertebrae are placed one over the other in such a way that there are small gaps on the sides through which the nerves can pass safely.

The intervertebral discs

The vertebral bodies are, in fact, not in direct contact with each other. They are separated by somewhat pliable but very strong discs. The discs act as shock absorbers: their structure would challenge even the best of engineers. They have a ring (annulus) surrounding a soft gelatinous centre (Fig. 13.5). The ring is made up of alternating layers of parallel tough collagen fibres. The arrangement of fibres produces a strong radial-ply effect. The small little disc can tolerate an amazingly heavy load without rupturing. The model that has been proposed for the intervertebral disc is that of a partially inflated football bladder placed between two flat pieces of wood (Fig. 13.6). If you would like to verify the strength of such a structure, get a football bladder, inflate it partially, close it tightly, and place it between two flat pieces of wood. Arrange for some restraint so that the bladder cannot slip out easily. Then stand on the structure: the structure may wobble, but the bladder will not burst. The disc does not even wobble because of the ring of tough radial-ply fibres. The result is that the disc cushions the load, spreads it evenly all over the surface of the disc, and also allows movement of the spine. The disc is so tough that when the spine is overloaded, it is more common for a vertebra to fracture than for a disc to rupture.

Disc prolapse

Slipped disc is a common expression but is a misnomer. Discs do not slip out of the intervertebral space. What actually happens is that chronic overloading or misuse of the back leads to wearing

The Poor Back 265

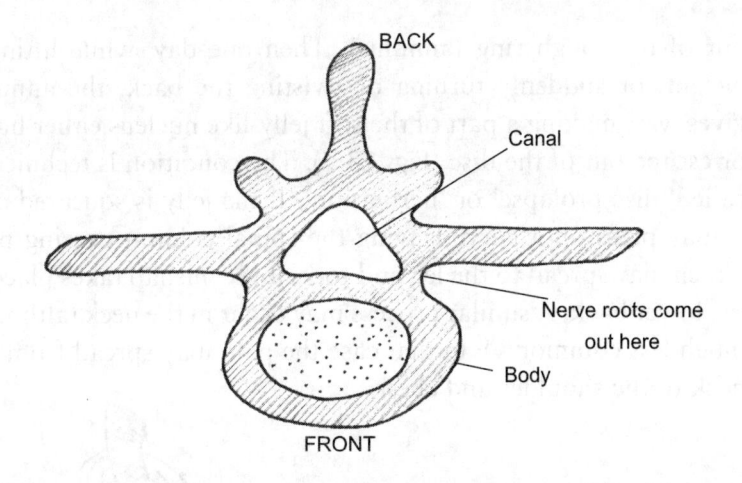

Fig. 13.4. *A diagrammatic sketch of a vertebra. The vertebral column has several such vertebrae, one on top of the other. The disc is interposed between the bodies of two neighbouring vertebrae. The spinal cord passes through the vertebral canal. The nerve roots emerge at the point indicated. At that point, the vertebrae are a little thin, and so moulded that two adjacent vertebrae form a hole on either side to accommodate the nerve roots.*

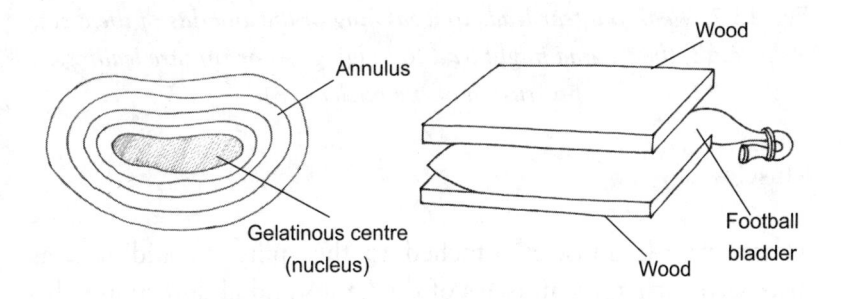

Fig. 13.5. *A diagrammatic sketch of an intervertebral disc.*

Fig. 13.6. *A model with the functional properties of an intervertebral disc.*

out of the tough ring (annulus). Then one day, while lifting a weight, or suddenly turning or twisting the back, the annulus gives way, making a part of the soft jelly-like nucleus either bulge or escape out of the disc (Fig. 13.7). The condition is technically called 'disc prolapse' or 'herniation'. If the jelly is squeezed out, it may press on a nerve leaving the spinal column causing pain which may spread to the leg and foot, if the mishap takes place in the lower back. A similar process may occur in the neck (although much less commonly): in that case the pain may spread from the neck to the shoulder and chest.

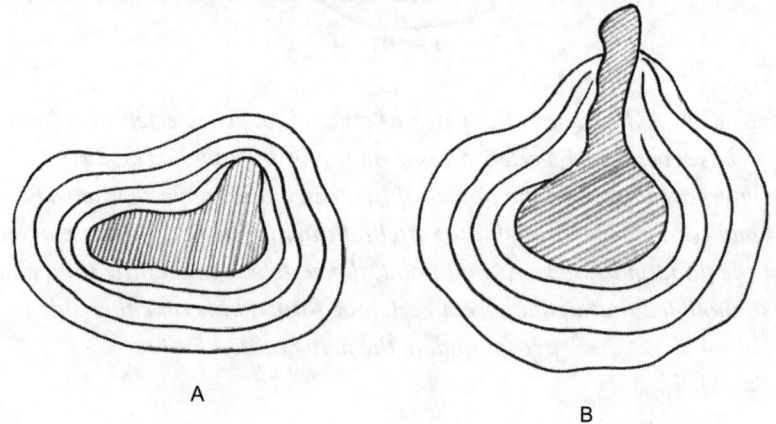

Fig. 13.7. *Wear and tear leads to weakning of the annulus of the discs. As a result, the trauma might lead to bulging (A) or rupture leading to protrusion of the nucleus (B).*

Muscles

There are 140 muscles attached to the spine. In addition, as discussed earlier, the muscles of the flanks and abdomen are also relevant to the health of the back. Similarly, shoulder, hip and even leg muscles have a direct or indirect relationship with the back. The strength, flexibility and balance of all these muscles is essential for a healthy back. By balance of muscles is meant the balance between the muscles which bend the back forwards (flexors) and those which bend it backwards (extensors). The strength of flexors and extensors should be well-matched.

We have already discussed how the contraction of muscles of the back, abdomen and flanks share the weight imposed on the back and thus protect it. The protection is so important that even when a backache seems to be due to a demonstrable defect in the bones or the disc, the root cause may be the muscles. Weakness of the muscles would prevent them from sharing the load on the spine adequately. That, in turn, would overload the vertebrae and discs, thereby increasing the chances of damaging them. The role of muscles also explains another paradox. Sometimes the age-related degenerative changes in the bones or discs are minimal, but the backache is severe. On the other hand, in some cases the degenerative changes are considerable, but there is no pain. This happens because the pain is actually due to weak muscles, but the weakness of the muscles does not show in X-rays. Therefore, the attention gets focused on degenerative changes, which are incidental, but get blamed for the pain. Another person with more pronounced age-related changes may have no pain if his muscles are strong.

Muscles are not only the commonest source of backaches, they are also the major site of backaches because the majority of pain-sensitive structures (receptors) of the back are located in the muscles. Sore muscles are usually the result of muscle spasm. A spasm is the prolonged uninterrupted contraction of muscles. Such a muscle consumes more energy than a relaxed muscle. As a by-product of greater energy use, it also produces more waste products such as carbon dioxide and lactic acid. On the other hand, the blood flow through a contracted muscle is less because of the squeezing effect of the contraction. Poor blood flow coupled with increased production of waste products leads to their accumulation in the muscle. The waste products stimulate pain-sensitive receptors in the muscle, leading to pain.

The spasm of back muscles may develop in at least two ways. First, an injury to the back (which may be accidental or may be due to weak muscles) leads to spasmodic contraction of muscles around the injury. The contraction serves a protective function by reducing the mobility of the injured structures. The contraction leads to pain, which is also protective because it further reduces the mobility. But protective or not, it is pain all the same. Secondly, mental tension induces muscle spasm even in the absence of injury. This is a reflection of the mind-body connection. When the mind is tense, the muscles also become tense. Stress-induced tension of the neck muscles often leads to pain in the neck and headaches. Similarly, stress-induced tension of the back muscles may lead to backaches. Furthermore, what happens is that a tense back becomes rigid, and a rigid back is more susceptible to injury (just as the rigid trunk of a tree might break in strong wind whereas the thinner but more pliable branches bend rather than break). If the rigid back is injured, the surrounding muscles undergo further spasmodic contraction, which in turn leads to more pain (Fig. 13.8).

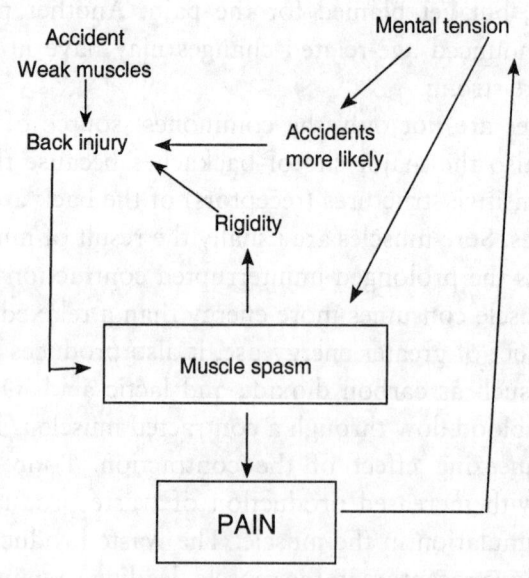

Fig. 13.8. *The complex relationship between mental tension, muscle spasm and back pain.*

The take-home message of the above discussion is that, contrary to commonsense, backache is basically not a problem of the backbone, but of the muscles attached to the backbone. Strong muscles are essential for preventing backache. And, when backache does occur, muscles are the major site of pain. Therefore, the treatment also requires relaxing, stretching and strengthening the muscles rather than fixing the bones.

Ligaments

Ligaments are band-like structures of high tensile strength fixed to bones. They restrict the movement of the joints to safe limits. However, ligaments are stretchable upto a point, and thus permit the necessary movement. The stretchability of ligaments can be maintained and improved upon by regular stretching exercises like yogic postures. The large number of ligaments in the back is important to its health, and injury to the ligaments is sometimes the root cause of back pain.

ACUTE AND CHRONIC BACK PAIN

An attack of acute back pain might be triggered by:
a. a major accident in which muscles or ligaments may get overstretched, or vertebrae may fracture, or an intervertebral disc might herniate,
b. a minor accident, like bending down to pick up a pen, or turning to talk to a friend: in these cases, some silent damage or muscle weakness is already present; the accident is only an 'excuse' – something like the proverbial last straw that broke the (already overloaded) camel's back, or
c. apparently nothing: here the cause may be the sudden spasm of muscles and/or the blood vessels supplying them, which may be precipitated by mental tension, exposure to cold, etc. The mechanism is similar to that which triggers a heart attack, but since a 'back attack' is not life-threatening, it is not called so.

Back pain might become chronic if:
a. an acute attack is treated with too long a bed rest or the excessive use of a lumbar support (belt), because both these can weaken the muscles.
b. an acute attack is treated with inadequate or inappropriate exercises.
c. the acute attack is due to an injury to a ligament. Ligaments heal poorly, and once injured, remain prone to repeated injury.

IS IT THE DISC?

Every back pain is not due to the slipped disc – in fact, most of the time it is muscles and other soft tissues. Some of the characteristics of disc pain are:

1. Initially it gets worse in spite of bed rest. It is after a few days or weeks that it starts getting better.
2. The person has great difficulty in putting on socks. He may find it easier to put on socks while lying down.
3. The pain increases on standing, and is relieved by lying down. Sitting is even worse than standing.
4. The pain increases during coughing, sneezing, laughing or straining.
5. The pain spreads to the buttocks, thighs and legs.
6. The pain has a tendency to become recurrent.

IS BACK PAIN A LIFESTYLE DISEASE?

It is quite clear from the above discussion that back pain is neither primarily a disease of bones or the disc, nor is it necessarily the result of a severe trauma. Let us now see how it is a lifestyle disease. Science and technology have given so many labour-saving gadgets to us that today our muscles do not have to work much and therefore remain weak. Weak muscles of the back and abdomen predispose us to back pain. Further, these weak muscles are inappropriately used while sitting for too long, without a break, in poorly designed chairs or car seats. And, when we do decide to take a break, we go on a holiday with heavy luggage, which may include some equipment for sports. Carrying the heavy luggage and playing strenuous games suddenly expose the weak muscles to loads to which they are not accustomed. Therefore, instead of coming back stronger, we may return from the holiday with a back injury. Sedentary life and overeating together promote obesity. And, obesity also increases the chances of back pain by overloading the spine. Apart from sedentary life, a major component of the modern lifestyle is mental stress. And, we have seen how stress is related to back pain (Fig. 13.8). Finally, smoking, a lifestyle factor too, also increases the risk for back pain, possibly by reducing blood flow to the back.

NECK PAIN

Neck pain is similar to low back pain in many ways. It is associated with sedentary work and poor posture. Keeping the neck bent forwards while working with books and doing paperwork, or while working on a computer sitting in a poorly designed seat, is inviting neck pain. Further, mental stress leads to the spasm of the neck and shoulder muscles. Age-related degenerative changes in the neck vertebrae (cervical spine) may be accelerated by these lifestyle factors, as in the case of the lower back (lumbar spine). These degenerative changes might lead to pressure on nerves issuing from the cervical spine, thereby leading to pain in the shoulder, near the shoulder blade or in the arms. In some cases, there might be a tingling sensation or weakness in the arms. The principles of the treatment of neck pain are also the same as those of back pain.

PREVENTION OF BACK PAIN

Prevention is not only better but also easier than the cure as far as back pain is concerned. Back pain is largely preventable, but requires a little effort and some precautions in daily life. Some of the most important measures for the prevention of back pain have been listed below.

1. Practise yogic postures everyday. Those particularly relevant to prevention of backache are *setubandhasana* and *pavanmuktasana, uttanapadasana* and *naukasana, pashchimottanasana* and *konasana, vajrasana* and *shashankasana, ushtrasana* and *parvatasana, bhujangasana* and *shalabhasana, trikonasana* and *ardhakatichakrasana*. The list is rather long, and perhaps all asanas listed in Chapter 1 could be listed here because, as discussed earlier, the back is intimately related not only to the muscles of the back and abdomen, but also to those of the shoulders and legs.
2. While the above postures are important, warming up before these postures, and relaxation between the postures, should not be neglected. Without the warm-up and relaxation, the asanas might occasionally lead to injury due to overstretching.
3. Yogic postures improve flexibility rather than strength. Normally they are enough for preventing backache. But if someone also wants very strong muscles, then he might add some strengthening exercises to yogic postures. Strengthening exercises involve repetitive movement against resistance.
4. Walk for about half an hour regularly. Walking exercises most of the muscles relevant to the prevention of back pain. One should walk consciously – becoming aware of the leg-back connection, and admiring the act of walking erect as a marvel of nature. We normally take the simple act of walking for granted – a person who cannot walk can tell us what a wonderful achievement it is.
5. While walking, wear comfortable shoes: high heels are out. The ideal is to wear sports shoes which support the arch of the foot adequately.

6. Avoid accidents. The floor at home and the workplace should be clean, dry and a little rough, lighting should be adequate, there should be no overcrowding due to excess furniture, etc, and if one deals with machinery, it should be handled with due precautions. However, one cannot control all these factors. Occasionally, we will have to walk on a highly polished or wet and slippery floor or walk through crowded spaces. When an accident takes place in some of these situations, it is not always simply an accident. It may occur because the person was walking at one place, but was mentally at another place. Thinking and doing too many things at the same time, mental stress, worry and preoccupations, are often behind what looks like an accident. To prevent these mishaps, one should cultivate the habit of doing everything with full attention.
7. Cultivate the right posture. One should sit or stand erect (but not tense).
8. If one stands for very long, one should keep shifting the weight from one leg to the other periodically. During prolonged standing, do not hesitate to use a back support, if available.
9. Sitting is even more unkind to the back than standing. If the work involves sitting, stand up and walk for a few minutes periodically. The seat should be firm (neither hard nor too soft), and should have a lumbar support at the right level for the individual (Fig.13.9).
10. While reading a book, keep it in such a way as to avoid excessive forward bending of the neck (Fig. 13.10).
11. While driving, use a car with a well-designed seat. Further, keep the seat forward so that the knees are raised a little above the seat.
12. Avoid long and frequent road journeys, specially on rough roads, in buses or trucks. Besides the posture and a possibly poorly-designed seat, the vibration in such journeys is bad for the back. That is why bus and truck drivers are specially

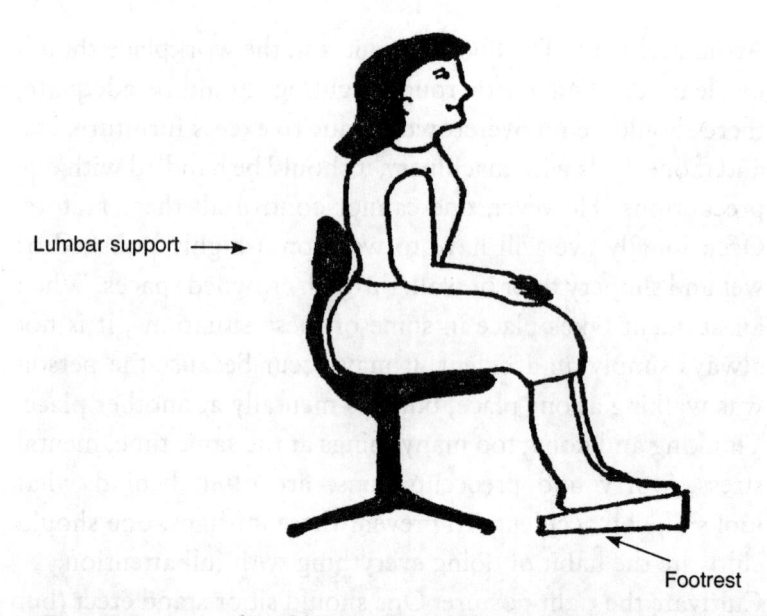

Fig. 13.9. *A comfortable seat should have a lumbar support which should fit closely the lumbar hollow of the person using the seat. A foot rest also helps by raising the knees a little bit so that the seat does not press too hard against the thighs. The person should sit with the back erect, the neck as erect as possible, and use a support for the arms and hands, specially if working on a computer.*

prone to backache. If a long journey by road is unavoidable, securing additional lumbar support by using a 'belt' (such belts are available with chemists) is worthwhile.

13. Sleep on a firm bed. Sleep either on the back, or on the side. Do not sleep on the tummy.
14. If possible, lie down in the afternoon after lunch for fifteen to thirty minutes. That may not be enough for an afternoon nap, but it helps the back. Becoming horizontal in the afternoon breaks the day into three parts of eight hours each instead of two parts consisting of eight hours of sleep (horizontal posture) and sixteen hours of wakefulness (vertical posture). That is a big difference. The back can tolerate eight hours of vertical posture much better than sixteen. During the

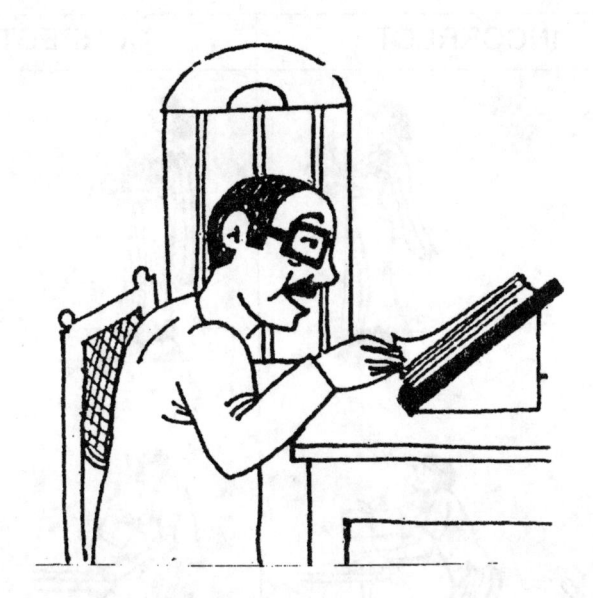

Fig. 13.10. *While reading, it is better to keep the book at an angle than to bend the neck.*

short afternoon 'stretching', the intervertebral discs get an opportunity to decompress and get ready for another eight hours of compression in the vertical posture.

15. Lift heavy objects with care. The correct way to lift weights is to keep the weight as close to the body as possible. The back should be bent a little backwards, not forwards. And, while initially picking up the object, do not stoop forwards. Use the legs instead to accomplish the job (Fig. 13.11). Finally, do not lift a weight beyond your capacity. If several objects have to be carried, it is better to carry a smaller number at a time and make more trips than to overdo in order to economise on the number of trips. Travel light. Further, carry a larger number of light units rather than a single heavy unit. Lift weights with full consciousness to avoid accidents due to sudden and jerky movements. An accident while lifting a weight can injure the back badly. Start lifting a weight in a premeditated manner.

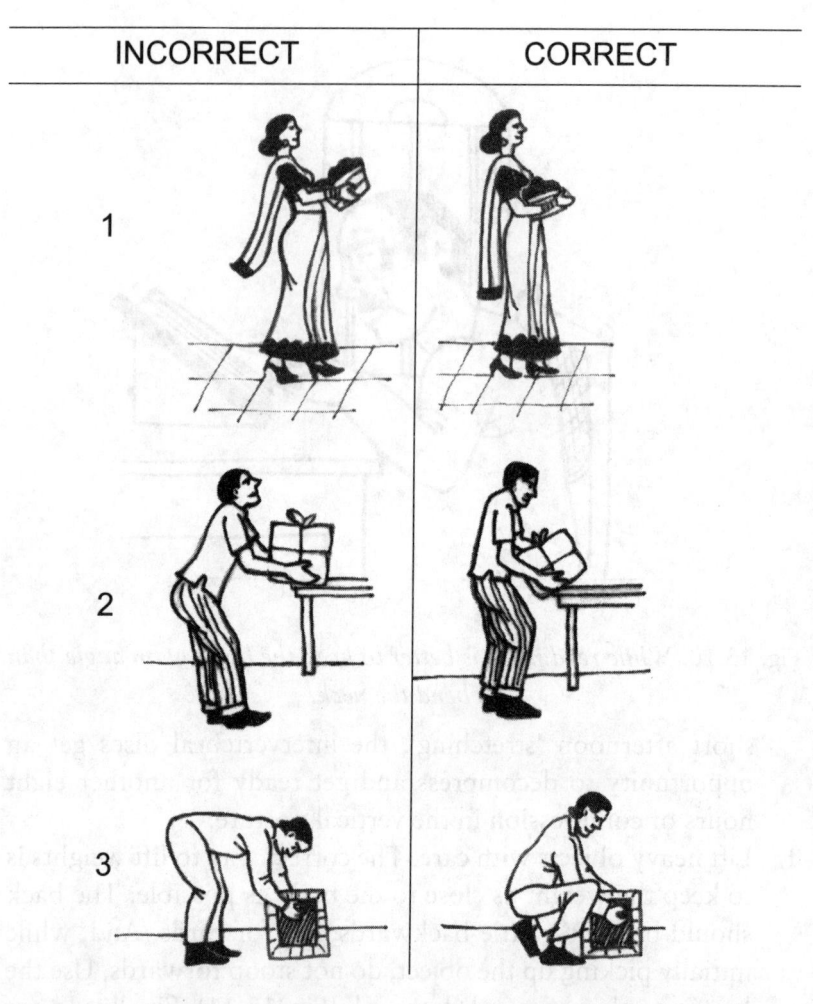

Fig. 13.11. *Incorrect and correct postures:*

1. *While carrying a typewriter, it would be incorrect to keep the heavier end of the load away from the body, and to stoop forwards.*
2. *While lifting a weight from a table, it is better to move as close to the weight as possible, bend the back a little backwards, and fold the legs a bit, and straighten them as the weight is lifted.*
3. *While lifting a weight from the ground, perform part of the sitting movement, and lift the load up with the legs.*

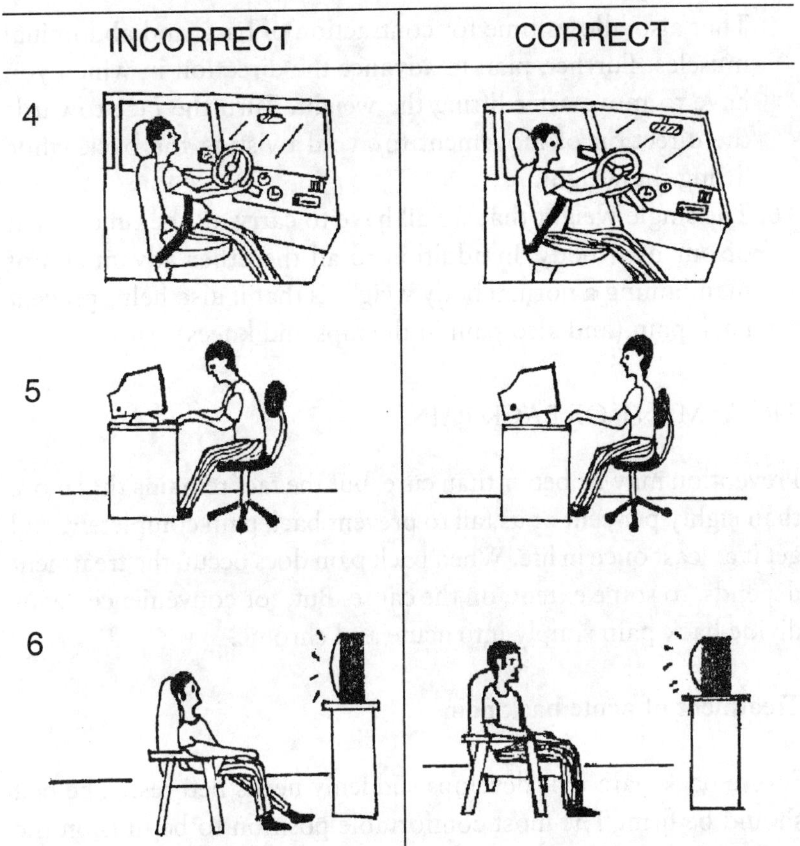

	INCORRECT	CORRECT
4		
5		
6		

Fig. 13.11. *Incorrect and correct postures (contd)*

4. *While driving, keep the car seat forward, the knees a little raised away from the seat. The car seat should have a well-fitting lumbar support*
5. *While working at the computer, sit erect, have the screen at the eye level, and use a chair with a well fitting lumbar support (the bulge in the back of the chair should fit well into your lumbar hollow).*
6. *While watching TV, do not sit on a very soft sofa with the back bent. Sit erect on a firm seat with a good lumbar support. If the back of the sofa is too far back, use an additional cushion at the back.*

That also allows time for contraction of back and abdominal muscles. Further, plan in advance the direction in which you have to move after lifting the weight. Turn the face towards the direction of movement to avoid twisting the back while lifting the weight.
16. The single weight that we all have to carry all the time is that of our own body. In addition to all the other advantages of maintaining a normal body weight is that it also helps prevent back pain (and also pain in the hips and knees).

TREATMENT OF BACK PAIN

Prevention may be better than cure, but the fact remains that more than eighty per cent of us fail to prevent back pain completely, and get it at least once in life. When back pain does occur, the treatment depends, to some extent, on the cause. But, for convenience, let us divide back pain simply into acute and chronic.

Treatment of acute back pain

Severe back pain that develops suddenly needs bed rest. The bed should be firm. The most comfortable position to be in is on the back, with a pillow kept under the knees (so that the legs stay a little bent without any effort). For a change in posture, lying on the side is also allowed, but while changing from one posture to the other, care should be taken to avoid twisting the spine. For a couple of days, one may avoid getting up even to eat or drink, but going cautiously to the toilet is generally allowed. Bed rest may be required for a few days to a few weeks, but if the pain does not improve substantially within two weeks, a thorough check-up is called for.

Exercises

It may seem paradoxical to talk of exercises along with bed rest. But a few simple exercises which can be done lying down should be started as early as possible during the period of bed rest itself. Some exercises are possible on the first or second day of the pain. Exercises appropriate for acute back pain, based on the recommendations of Swami Vivekananda Kendra, Prashanti Kuteeram, Bangalore, have been described below. These exercises should be continued till other exercises described later are possible.

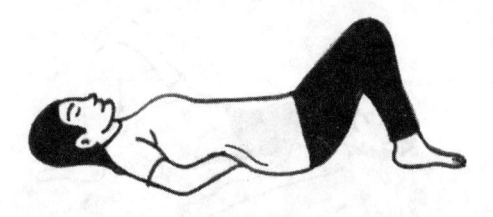

Prressing the spine

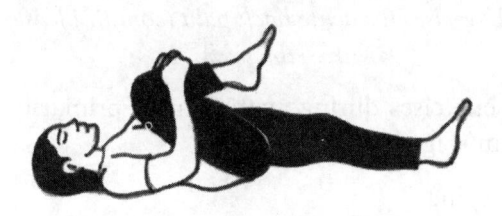

Folded leg lumbar stretch (one leg)

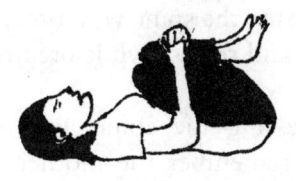

Folded leg lumbar stretch (both leg)

Fig. 13.12. Exercises for acute back pain

Dorsal stretch

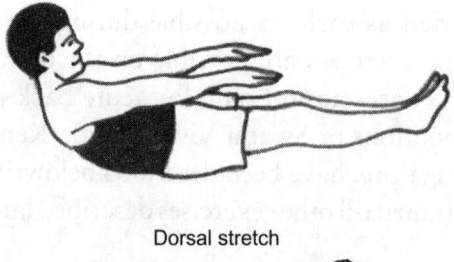

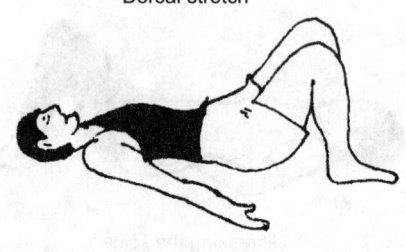

Shavasana, with legs folded

Fig. 13.12. *Exercises for acute back pain (contd). Please see details in the text.*

The aim of exercises during acute pain is primarily to relax the muscle spasm (Fig. 13.12).

Pressing the spine

Lie down on the back and fold the legs. Press the spine against the bed, keep it pressed for a few seconds, and release. Repeat five times.

Next, synchronise pressing the spine with breathing. Press the spine while breathing out, and release while breathing in. Repeat five times.

Next, synchronise pressing the spine with breathing and chanting. It is natural to remember the mother when in pain. When breathing out, press the spine against the bed and chant 'maaa…'. While breathing in, relax. Feel the soothing vibrations of the chant. Repeat five times.

In this exercise, a small folded towel might be kept under the painful part of the spine. For further comfort, hands might be inserted between the towel and the back, the palms facing the towel.

Folded-leg lumbar stretch

This exercise might aggravate the pain; in that case, one can wait for a day or two before trying it.

Keep the left leg straight, and bend the right leg. Slowly bring the right knee closer to the chest using both hands with their fingers interlocked (as in *pavanmuktasana*). Do not raise the head. Keep the right knee pressed against the chest for a few seconds, and then straighten the leg to return to the starting position. Repeat five times. Then repeat five times with the other leg. Next, repeat five times with both legs together.

Then repeat the whole cycle five times, synchronising the movements with the breathing: breathe out while pressing the knee(s) against the chest; breathe in while straightening the leg(s).

Finally, repeat the whole cycle, synchronising the movements with breathing and chanting. Chant 'maaa…' when breathing out, and feel the soothing vibrations of the chant. Repeat five times.

Dorsal stretch

This is still more difficult, and one might have to wait another few days till the pain subsides a bit.

Lie down on the back with the legs straight. Raise the upper part of the body, keeping the arms horizontal and the palms facing downwards. Come down slowly and return to the starting position. Repeat five times.

Synchronise the above movements with breathing: breathe out while raising the body, breathe in while coming down. Repeat five times.

Finally, synchronise the above movements with breathing, and chant 'maaa…' while breathing out. Feel the soothing vibrations of the chant. Repeat five times.

Relaxation

After the exercises, relax for five minutes in *shavasana*. Breathe slowly: as you breathe in, the abdomen moves out, and as you breathe out, the abdomen moves in. You may chant 'maaa...' silently as you breathe out.

The above set of exercises for acute back pain should be done 4-5 times per day, with an interval of 2-3 hours between two consecutive sessions.

N.B. The entire range of exercises, and the number of repetitions mentioned here, are not sacrosanct. Listen to your body: you may stop when you feel you have stepped out of your comfort zone.

Rest as an opportunity to reflect

The enforced bed rest might be looked upon as an opportunity to reflect on your life, your goals, and the direction in which you are going. You might discover that you need a mid-course correction which is within your reach.

Meditation and visualisation

Meditate while lying down in bed. Towards the end of meditation, visualise the Mother, a loved one, or someone who represents to you the Divine in a human form, caressing your back with his/her hands. Feel the love and healing power of the touch. Visualise your back getting healed and remain in the blissful state for a few minutes. Repeat 3-4 times a day at a few hours interval.

Cold/hot fomentation

In general, after an injury (to the back or elsewhere), cold fomentation is beneficial up to the first 48 hours after the injury – the sooner it is started, the better. After 48 hours, hot fomentation is more effective.

Drugs

Pain killers and muscle relaxants are the drugs used for acute back pain. If all the above measures are taken, one should need only the minimal dose of these drugs, if at all, to stay comfortable in spite of back pain.

Follow-up action

After the acute pain subsides, the exercises and other measures recommended for chronic back pain should be adopted to prevent further episodes of acute back pain.

Treatment for chronic back pain

Chronic pain in the lower back is a common problem which can generally be managed satisfactorily by an appropriate exercise-based programme. Only a minority of patients need surgery. Dr Arthur Brownstein's programme, a programme of proven efficacy, consists of progressively difficult stretching exercises over a period of two months followed by strengthening exercises.

TABLE 13.1. SUGGESTED SCHEDULE OF YOGIC POSTURES FOR CHRONIC BACK PAIN*

Weeks 1-2

Prishthbhoomitadasana
Folded leg lumbar stretch (*Pavanmuktasana*, without raising the head)
Bhujangasana

Weeks 3-4

Add to the above:
Setubandhasana
Shalabhasana

Weeks 5-8

Add to the above:
Crossed-leg lumbar stretch
Vajrasana
Ushtrasana
Parvatasana
Dhanurasana
Ardhmatsyendrasana
Trikonasana/Ardhakatichakrasana

Week 9 onwards

Add to the above:
Prasarit Padahastasana (*Padahastasana*, with feet about one foot apart)

---

* Add relaxing postures between asanas and at the end of the session.

ASANAS FOR CHRONIC BACK PAIN

WEEKS 1-2

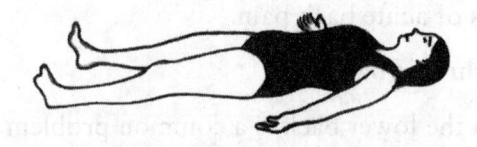

SHAVASANA
(The cadaveric posture)

Shavasana, a relaxing posture. One should lie down with feet apart, hands away from the body, palms facing upwards, with the eyes closed, and breathe slowly and deeply. As the air goes in, the abdomen goes up and as the air is breathed out, the abdomen comes down. The whole body should be relaxed completely and the mind should be at peace.

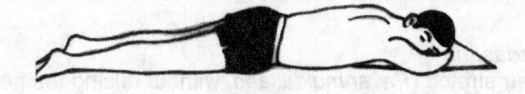

MAKARASANA
(The crocodile posture)

Makarasana, a posture particularly suitable for relaxing between asanas which are performed with the belly touching the ground, such as bhujangasana and dhanurasana.

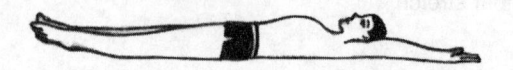

PRISHTHBHOOMITADASANA
(Stretching, lying down)

Fig. 13.13. Exercises for chronic back pain

The Poor Back   285

WEEKS 1-2 (contd.)

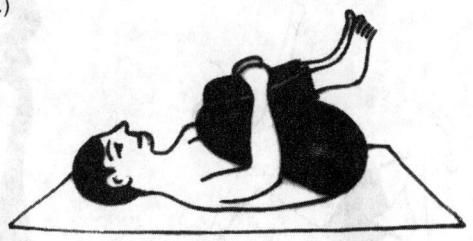

PAVANMUKTASANA (Without raising the head)
(Folded leg lumbar stretch)

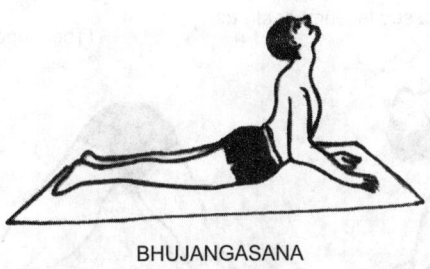

BHUJANGASANA
(The cobra posture)

WEEKS 3-4

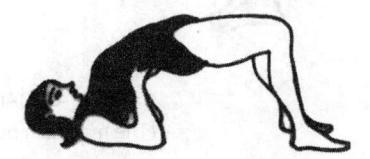

SETUBANDHASANA
(The bridge posture)

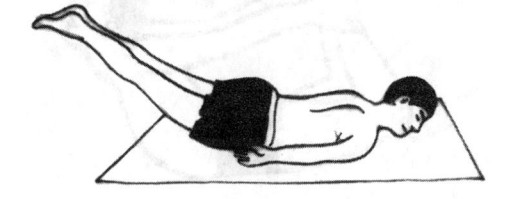

SHALABHASANA
(The locust posture)

Fig. 13.13. Exercises for chronic back pain (contd)

WEEKS 5-8

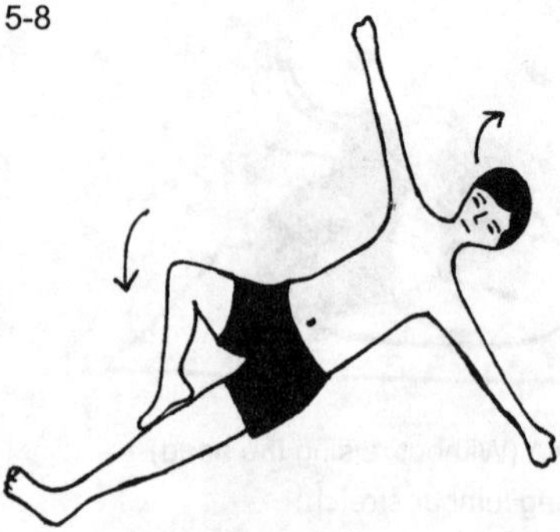

Crossed leg lumbar stretch

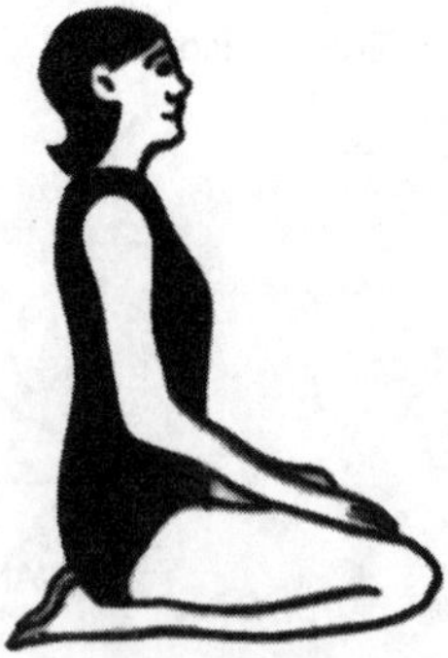

VAJRASANA
(The thunderbolt posture)

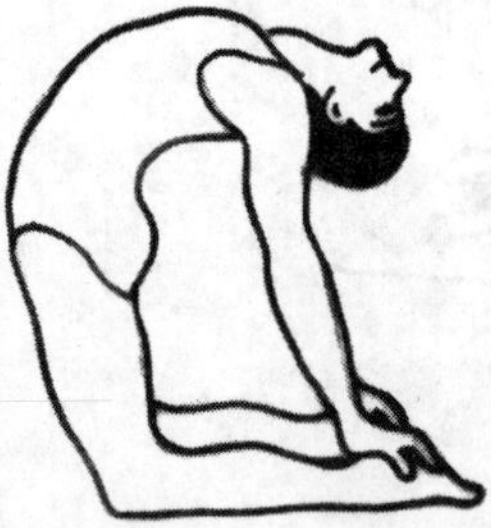

USHTRASANA
(The camel posture)

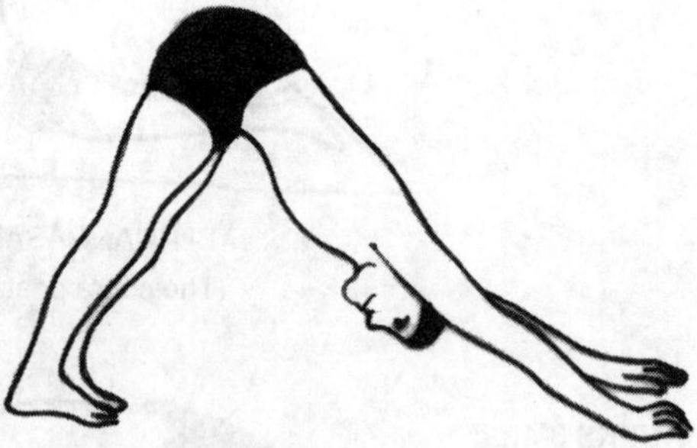

PARVATASANA
(The mountain posture)

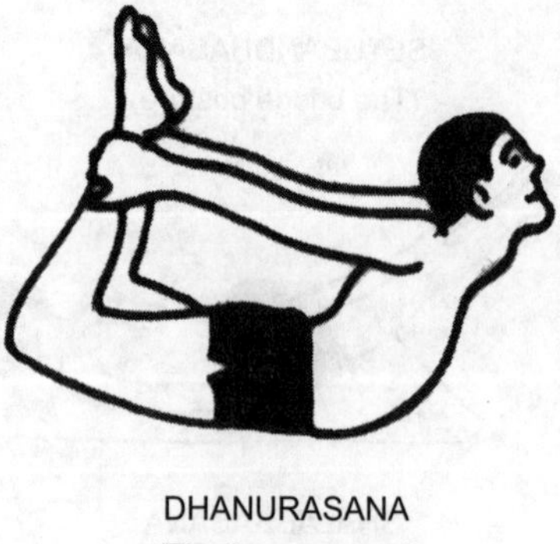

DHANURASANA
(The bow posture)

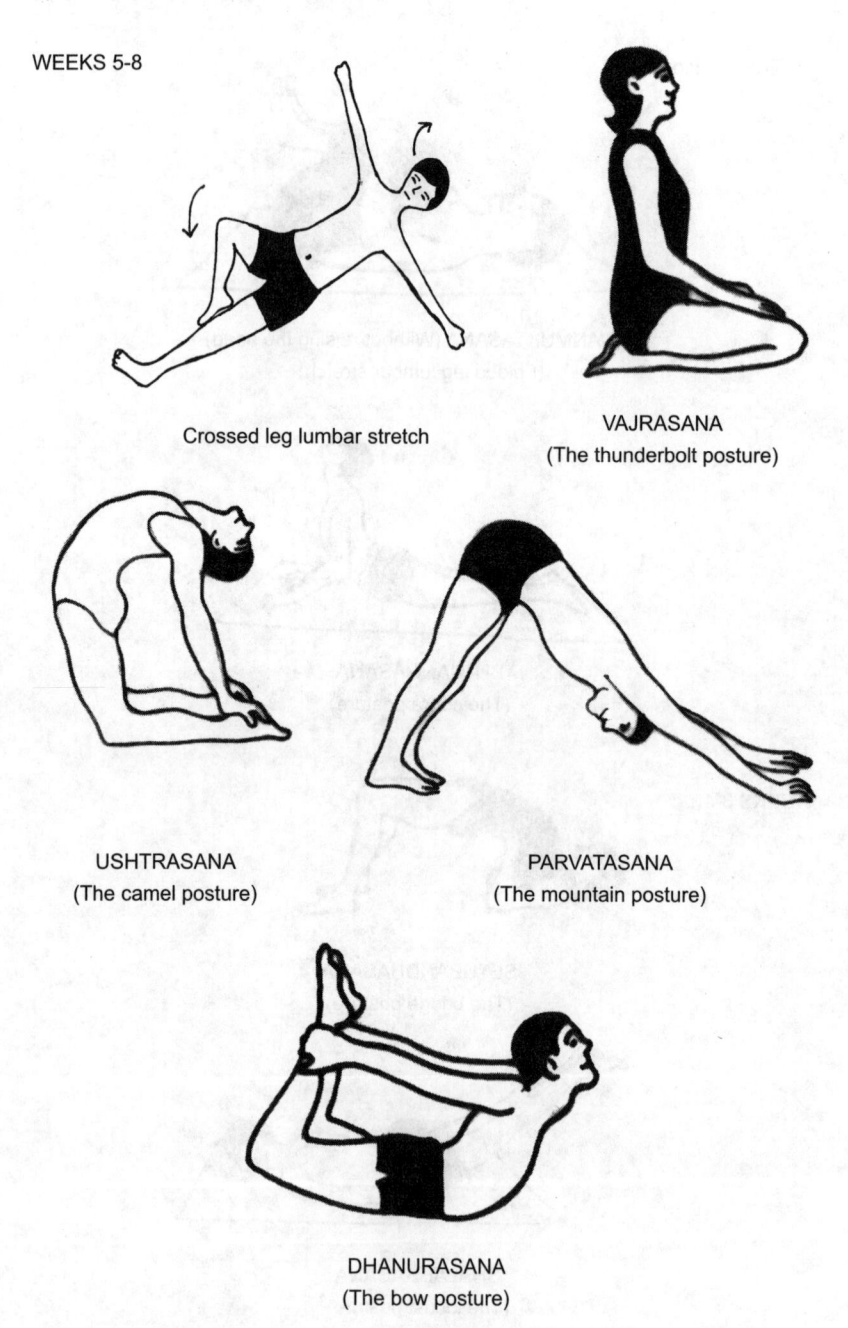

Fig. 13.13. *Exercises for chronic back pain (contd).*

WEEKS 5-8 (contd.)

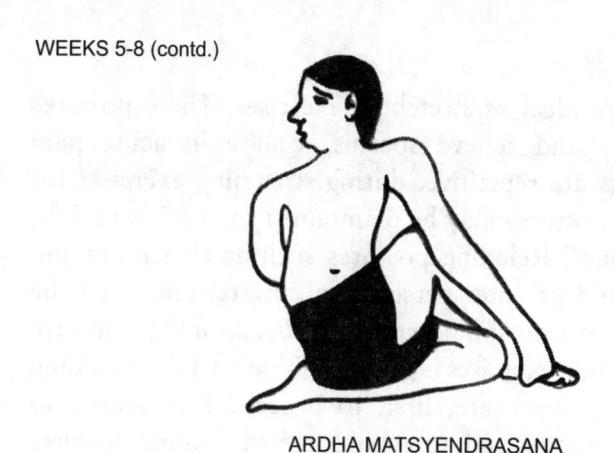

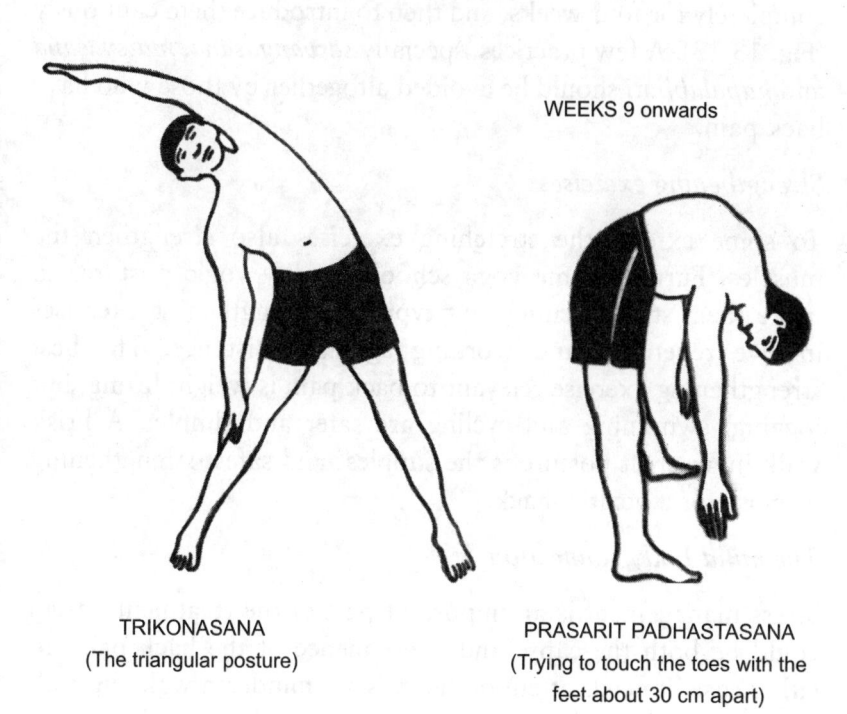

ARDHA MATSYENDRASANA

WEEKS 9 onwards

TRIKONASANA
(The triangular posture)

PRASARIT PADHASTASANA
(Trying to touch the toes with the feet about 30 cm apart)

Fig. 13.13. *Exercises for chronic back pain (contd). Please see details in the text. Also consult Chapter 1 and Appendix 1 to determine the sequence of the postures.*

Stretching exercises

Yogic postures are ideal as stretching exercises. These postures achieve flexibility and relieve spasms. Unlike in acute pain where movements are repetitive, during stretching exercises for chronic pain, the postures may be maintained for 10-20 seconds, and done only once. Relaxing postures such as *shavasana* and *makarasana* should be interspersed appropriately between the postures, and the session should end with *shavasana*. A tentative schedule of stretching exercises is given in Table 13.1. The guiding principles of the scheme are, first, to proceed from easier to difficult postures; and second, to avoid forward bending postures completely for four weeks, and then to introduce them cautiously (Fig. 13.13). A few practices, specially *sarvangasana*, *matsyasana* and *kapalabhati* should be avoided altogether by those who have back pain.

Strengthening exercises

To some extent, the stretching exercises also strengthen the muscles. Further, some yoga schools modify yogic postures to make them strengthening. But typically, strengthening exercises involve repetition and working against resistance. The best strengthening exercise relevant to back pain is weight lifting, but jogging, swimming and cycling are safer and simpler. A brisk walk in an erect posture is the simplest and safest strengthening exercise for a healthy back.

The mind-body connection

Stress management is an important part of the treatment. Stress could be both the cause and consequence of the back pain. In either case, it needs attention. Pain is a reminder, a wake-up call, which alerts the patient to take a fresh look at his life. The patient may discover that in the process of pursuing material progress he has forgotten the simple pleasures of life such as looking at the sunrise, or listening to the birds sing. Or, he may resolve bottled-up anger against someone, which has taken away his peace and equanimity. The pain may give the person an opportunity to rediscover virtues such as love, compassion and forgiveness. The warmth of these positive emotions can dissolve the negative emotions, and restore the peace of mind. Thus pain itself becomes a channel for breaking the vicious cycle of stress and pain.

Meditation and visualisation, as described under acute back pain, are beneficial also for chronic pain.

Intractable back pain

Sometimes the back pain just refuses to go away. In such cases, the poor back has been subjected to just about everything possible in an attempt to relieve pain: freezing cold or heat – superficial or deep; rest or exercise; diathermy; corsets; ultrasound; infrared rays; hydrotherapy; electrical stimulation; manipulation; traction; epidural injections; biofeedback; acupuncture; and of course, surgery, sometimes repeated up to three times. Naturally, to discuss such cases is beyond the scope of this book. But two factors which might contribute to the pain becoming intractable need attention: rest and corsets (belts).

Too much bed rest, beyond what is necessary, without any exercises for the back, weakens the muscles. The reason is simple: muscles not used for a prolonged period grow weak. While lying down, hardly any muscles are used. Therefore, the muscles of the back, abdomen as well as the limbs grow weak. And, we have seen how weak muscles can themselves encourage back pain.

Similarly, the frequent use of lumbar supports/corsets (belts) also makes the action of muscles unnecessary. A situation in which normally the back and abdominal muscles would contract to protect the spine can pass peacefully without muscular contraction if the person is using a belt. Thus these muscles get weak through not being used, and make the back pain persistent.

In short, the use of prolonged bed rest and belts should be judicious. Appropriate exercises should be started as soon as possible. Normal daily activity should also be resumed early.

If up to two weeks of bed rest does not help, one should not simply go on extending bed rest in the hope that more rest will by itself improve the situation. Instead, in such situations, a thorough search for the underlying cause of back pain is called for. Prolonging the bed rest or excessive use of the belt might unwittingly prolong the pain and make it intractable.

TREATMENT OF NECK PAIN

As mentioned earlier, the causes of neck pain are analogous to those of back pain. The principles of treatment are also similar.

Treatment of acute pain

For neck pain, bed rest is not necessary, but restricting the movements of the neck is helpful. This happens automatically because the movements are painful. Further, pain induces muscle spasm, thereby making the muscles rigid. Rigid muscles stabilise the neck, which is good; but rigid muscles might also aggravate the pain. The solution is to spend some time on appropriate exercises which relax the muscles. Exercises appropriate for acute neck pain, based on the recommendations of Swami Vivekananda Kendra, Prashanti Kuteeram, Bangalore, have been described below.

Lie down flat with the back on the floor or a hard bed with a very thin mattress or carpet spread on it. Keep a folded towel under the neck, and pull its ends to bring them in front of your shoulders. By doing this, the towel will fill up the gap between the neck and the floor, and thus the neck will be well supported (Fig. 13.14). Now start the following exercises one by one:

Pressing the neck

Keep the legs straight, or bend them at the knees, whichever is more comfortable. Keep the arms straight, by the side of the body and close to it, the palms facing downwards. Close the eyes. Press the back of the head, neck and shoulders on the bed, hold for a few seconds and then release. Repeat five times.

Towel

Pressing the neck

Hands in and out breathing

Rolling the neck sideways

Hand stretch breathing

Shavasana with legs folded

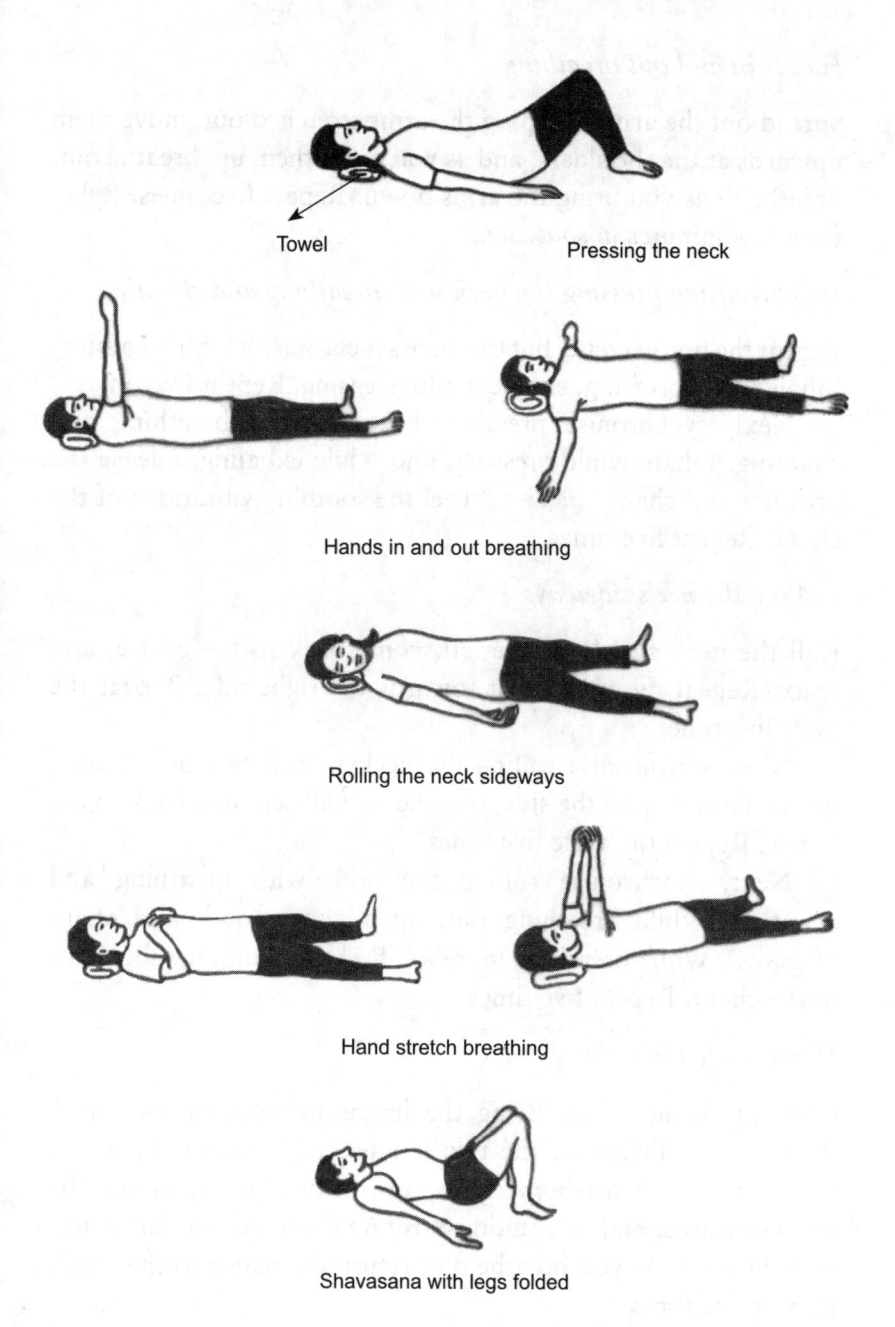

Fig. 13.14. *Exercises for acute neck pain. Please see details in the text.*

Hands in and out breathing

Spread out the arms. Keeping the arms stretched out, move them upwards at the shoulders, and as you move them up, breathe out. Breathe in as you bring the arms down. Repeat five times. Relax for a few minutes in *shavasana*.

Synchronising pressing the neck with breathing and chanting

Repeat the first exercise, but this time synchronise it with breathing. Inhale while pressing, exhale while releasing. Repeat five times.

Next, synchronise pressing the neck with breathing and chanting. Inhale while pressing, and while exhaling, release the pressure and chant 'maaa ...' Feel the soothing vibrations of the chant. Repeat five times.

Rolling the neck sideways

Roll the neck slowly to the left, come back to the centre, and relax. Repeat the movement towards the right side. Repeat the cycle five times.

Next, synchronise rolling the neck with breathing. Breathe out while rolling to the side, breathe in while coming back to the centre. Repeat the cycle five times.

Next, synchronise rolling the neck with breathing and chanting. While breathing out, open your mouth and chant 'maaa...'. While breathing in, relax. Feel the soothing vibrations of the chant. Repeat five times.

Hand stretch breathing

Continue lying down. Bring the hands in front of the chest. Interlock the fingers of the two hands, and place the hands so joined on the breast bone. Now, as you breathe in, stretch the arms upwards, and as you do so, rotate the hands so that palms face the roof. As you breathe out, return the hands to the chest. Repeat five times.

Relaxation

After the exercises, relax for five minutes in *shavasana*. Breathe slowly. As you breathe in, the abdomen moves out; and as you breathe out, the abdomen moves in. You may chant 'maaa..' silently as you breathe out.

The above set of exercises for acute neck pain may be done three times per day: morning, afternoon and evening. However, the number of exercises, and the number of repetitions mentioned here are not sacrosanct. Listen to your body: you may stop when you feel you have stepped out of your comfort zone.

As with back pain, neck pain may also be used as an opportunity to press the reset button of life. Meditation and visualisation may also be added to accelerate the process of healing. The principles of using hot fomentation and drugs are also similar to those for back pain. After the acute pain subsides, exercises recommended for chronic neck pain should be continued to prevent further episodes of acute back pain.

Treatment of chronic neck pain

Instead of concentrating on the neck, it is advisable to do almost all the exercises which a healthy person should do (Chapter 1) because a person with a neck also has a back, a heart, lungs, etc, to take care of. However, a few points may be kept in mind:

1. Lay greater emphasis on loosening exercises of the hands, elbows and shoulders.
2. Turn the neck up and down, bend it to the right and left, and turn it to the right and left, 8-10 times each, slowly and gently. The up and down movement should be specially gentle and cautious. Do not perform clock-wise and anti-clock-wise rotations of the neck unless permitted by your doctor or physiotherapist.

3. Avoid *sarvangasana* and *matsyasana*, and *kapalabhati*. These practices should be avoided by also those having back pain.

CLOSING THOUGHTS

Back pain is typically a middle-age problem, the age when one is passing through the busiest and most stressful period of one's life. At home, the children are growing up; on the work front, one's career is important; and it is still too early to avoid social and family commitments. In short, back pain attacks when one can afford it the least. However, getting worked up only makes matters worse: the stress adds to the pain. Instead, the pain can be looked upon as a blessing, a welcome excuse to relax, reassess priorities, and redirect life. No matter how important are the jobs pending, heavens will not fall and the world will not come to an end if they are not done by the person who has been forced to bed because of the pain. Important jobs get done anyhow by someone or the other. A good dictum in life is, take your work seriously, but do not take yourself seriously. With this attitude, the pain does not last long, and returning to work is no problem. Just as being obsessed with work is wrong, being obsessed with the pain is also wrong. If one likes work, returning to work is therapeutic. The experience of pain in the back helps in taking care of the posture, observing due precautions while lifting a weight, and asking for help if a job seems beyond one's physical capacity.

Fortunately, age is kind to the back. As one gets older, fresh episodes of acute back pain generally become less frequent.[1] It is partly because the spine becomes less flexible. A spine which is less flexible has a narrower range of movement, but is also less likely to be injured. Further, as a person gets older, he becomes less impulsive, movements become more measured and less jerky,

---

[1] The onset of persistent back pain in old age may be due to spread of cancer to the spine from the prostate or somewhere else in the body.

and the society expects less from him by way of physical work. The person is also less shy to ask for help, and is offered help more often, which he is quite willing to accept gratefully. The end result is a decline in prevalence of backache after the age of forty-five. But since nobody can reach that happy age without passing through the vulnerable period, we all need to know not to panic when back pain strikes.

Frequently Asked Questions

1. *Why does the back take two months or more to heal?*

    An injury to an organ damages or kills some of its cells. Healing involves repair of the damage, replacement of the damaged cells, and removal of the debris. The rate at which healing takes place depends on the inherent properties of the tissue involved, and is to some extent related to its blood supply. Cells of the oral mucosa (the membrane lining the inside of the mouth) divide very rapidly and replace dead cells promptly. Therefore, if the tongue gets burnt by a hot drink, the abnormal feeling in the tongue lasts hardly one day. But if the skin is burnt, it takes two weeks to heal. Muscles, tendons and ligaments, the tissues commonly damaged in those having back pain, take 2-3 months to heal. Further, the blood supply to tendons and ligaments is very poor. Therefore, they may not ever heal completely. What happens is that the dead cells, instead of getting replaced by tendon or ligament cells, might get replaced by fibrous tissue (a non-specific packing material). The result is that continuity is restored, but the healed area remains weak and vulnerable. That is why, a much milder injury might lead to a recurrence of the pain at exactly the same spot as before.

2. *What is sciatica?*

    Since nerve roots emerge from the spinal column, a variety of problems in the back might lead to compression or entrapment of the nerve roots. The roots most commonly involved are those in the lower back. The symptoms, commonly called sciatica, consist of pain in the buttocks, back of the thighs, the ankle and part of the foot. Depending on whether the pain or numbness affect the inside of the foot (specially the big toe) or the outside of the foot, the doctor can deduce which nerve root is involved. Different causes of sciatica can be distinguished from one another by finding out whether the pain is aggravated by coughing, whether the pain is relieved or worsened by lying down, etc.

3. *What is spondylosis?*

Spondylosis is a general term for changes in the vertebral column due to wear and tear. The wear and tear affects cartilage and discs. Cartilage is softer than bone. When it wears out, it is replaced by the bone. The rather bulky and ill-placed bony replacements are called osteophytes. Spondylosis commonly affects either the region around the neck (cervical spondylosis) or the lower back (lumbar spondylosis). Besides pain in the region of the spine affected, spondylosis may also give symptoms due to compression or irritation of the nerve roots issuing from that part of the spine.

4. *What is better: to sit erect without a backrest, or to sit in a well-designed chair having a backrest with lumbar support?*

Sitting erect is a good posture. It also involves some activity of thoracic, abdominal and back muscles, and therefore strengthens them. But sitting in even a good posture for too long will eventually be tiring, and the back may start aching. On the other hand, a backrest with lumbar support makes things easier by relieving the muscles. But not using the muscles weakens them.

Thus both the alternatives have pros and cons. The ideal

probably is to keep alternating between both. One may spend as much time without a backrest as comfortable, and then use the backrest. When the body feels adequately relaxed, one may again discontinue the use of the backrest. Further, one may also take a break from sitting whenever possible. Standing and walking relieve the strain of sitting because they are kinder to the lower back than sitting down.

A similar dilemma faces patients with back pain who have been prescribed a belt for lumbar support. The belt feels comfortable but also eliminates the need for contraction of back and abdominal muscles, thereby weakening the natural protection. The ideal again is to strike a balance: use the belt when necessary, but also be without it for some time to strengthen the muscles.

5. *Why are forward bending exercises avoided during back pain?*

There is a ligament that runs from the top to the bottom of the spine. Bending forward stretches this ligament, and might require it to lengthen by as much as thirty-five per cent. This amount of stretching of the ligament is not good for a painful back.

For Further Reading

Brownstein A, *Healing Back Pain Naturally.* Mumbai: Magna Publishing Co. Ltd., 2003.
Nagarathna R, Nagendra HR, *Yoga for Back Pain.* Bangalore: Swami Vivekananda Yoga Prakshana, 2001.
Porter R.W., *Management of Back Pain.* Edinburgh: Churchill Livingstone, 2nd Edition, 1993.

14

Gut Feelings

To eat is human; to digest, divine.

MARK TWAIN

The healthy gut works silently. On the other hand, one of the first signs of ill health is a gut that makes its presence felt. No wonder, gut feelings are a trusted indicator of how things are.

UNDERSTANDING THE GUT

When we swallow a morsel of food, it marks the beginning of a long journey which the food makes through the stomach and intestines (Fig. 14.1).[1] During this journey, food is mechanically crushed, chemically simplified (digested) and then transferred

---

[1] The scientific term for the entire 'tube' from the mouth to the anus is the alimentary canal. A more common term is the gastrointestinal tract (*gastro*, stomach), which makes up most of the alimentary canal. The specialists who treat diseases of the alimentary canal, liver and pancreas are called gastroenterologists (*entero*, intestine). Gut is a colloquial term used for the stomach, intestines and related structures.

across the intestinal wall into the blood (absorbed). It is only when food enters the blood that it is truly within the body. Food which is not absorbed is eventually discarded as faecal matter, and is therefore of no use to the body (Fig.14.2).

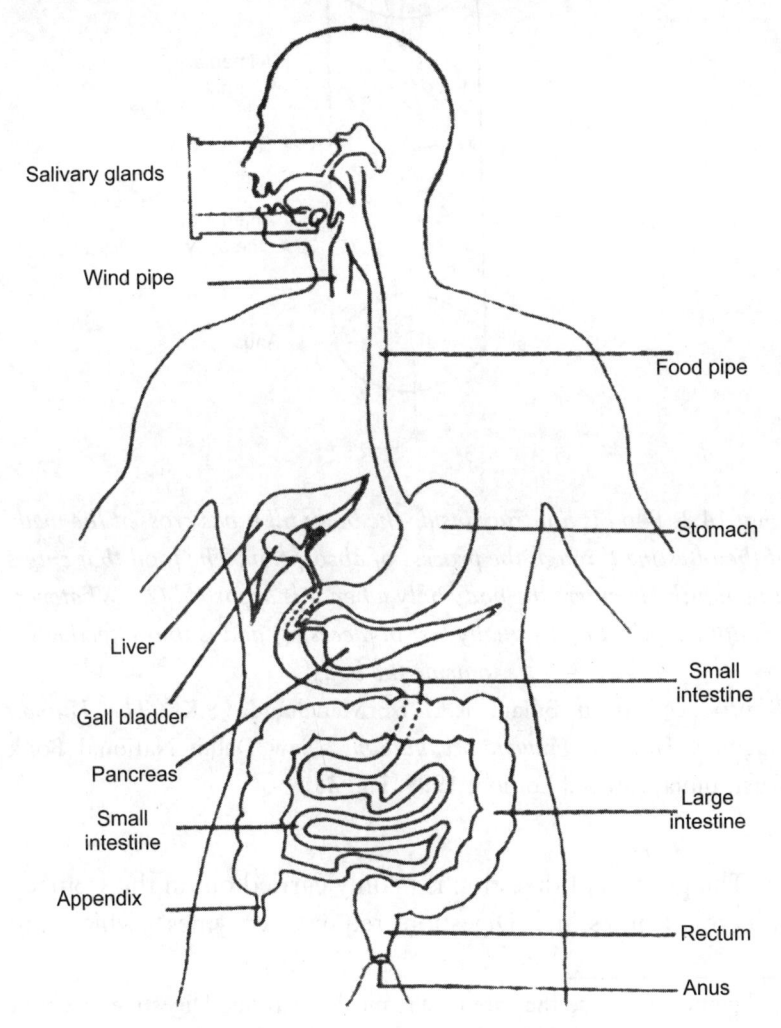

Fig. 14.1. *The digestive tract.*
(Reproduced from Bijlani R.L. & Manchanda S.K., *The Human Machine: How to prevent breakdowns.* New Delhi: National Book Trust, India, Revised Edition, 1999, Fig. 21)

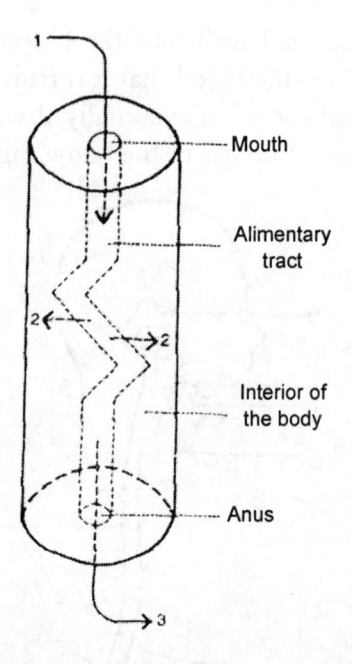

Fig. 14.2. *Food is not truly inside the body till it has crossed the wall of the intestine through the process of absorption. The food that enters the mouth (1) enters the body only when it is absorbed (2). Whatever is not absorbed is eventually lost in faeces (3) and is thus effectively outside the body.*
(Reproduced from Bijlani R.L. & Manchanda S.K., *The Human Machine: How to prevent breakdowns*. New Delhi: National Book Trust, India, Revised Edition, 1999, Fig. 25)

The process of digestion is mainly carried out in the stomach and small intestine. Digestion requires enzymes[2] which are

---

[2] Enzymes increase the rate of chemical reactions. Digestive enzymes break down complex nutrient molecules in food into their simpler units. Without the enzymes, the reactions involved in digestion would occur at a negligible rate, if at all, at the body temperature. Chemically, all enzymes are proteins.

present in juices manufactured by the stomach, small intestine and pancreas. Although the bile manufactured by the liver does not contain enzymes, bile is required for the digestion of fats. Secretions of the pancreas and liver are also delivered to the small intestine where they carry out their digestive functions. The process of absorption is mainly carried out in the small intestine.

Undigested and indigestible food cannot be absorbed: it is delivered to the large intestine. In the healthy gut, most of the residue delivered to the large intestine consists of dietary fibre. Part of this residue is fermented by the bacteria present in the large intestine. Fermentation produces gases. Part of the gases are absorbed into the blood; the remaining gases are passed as flatus. The residue that is not fermented reaches the terminal part of the large intestine, and is eventually evacuated as faecal matter. What goes on in the large intestine is, however, more than processing and disposal of waste. Apart from the contribution that some vitamins manufactured by the intestinal bacteria might be making to our nutrition, bacterial metabolism also produces some fatty acids which are important for colonic health. Some precious water and electrolytes are also absorbed in the large intestine. On the other hand, dietary fibre holds water and ensures that enough water is left behind for the stool to remain soft.

Not so simple

From what has been said above, one may get the impression that once the food has been swallowed, it just moves through ten metres of the gut, receives appropriate treatment in the right sequence, the nutrients are absorbed, and the residue is evacuated. The entire operation is too complex to be described so simply. It requires the secretion of various digestive juices at just the right time and place, and in the right quantity. Hence the secretion of the juices should get switched on and off appropriately. It is also necessary for the food to stay at one place to be treated adequately, and then to move on to the next section of the gut. Food cannot move by itself: it has to be propelled by the gut. Thus digestion and absorption are highly coordinated activities. Coordination is achieved in the body by the nervous and endocrine systems.[3] Besides being subject to the general influences of the nervous and endocrine systems, the gut has nerve cells and endocrine cells of its own.[4] The local nervous system of the gut and its endocrine cells interact, in turn, with the general nervous and endocrine systems. The nervous and endocrine systems mediate the effects of thoughts and emotions on the body. That is why healthy digestion depends so heavily on the mental state. The mere thought of appetising food makes the mouth water.[5] Panic makes a person rush to the toilet. Chronic anger and hostility might lead to a peptic ulcer. No wonder, digestive problems are among the commonest which take a person to a doctor. And, at least half of the patients going to gastroenterologists have either anxiety or depression.

HELPING THE GUT

If we help the gut by eating the right amount of the right type of food at the right time and in the right way, it works silently and efficiently. If the gut works well, we are well-nourished. That is why the health of the gut mirrors the general health of an individual.

Just as the gut mirrors the health of the whole body, the health of the gut depends on our lifestyle as a whole, not just on what we eat. However, the focus in this chapter will be only on those

---

[3] The endocrine system secretes hormones. Hormones are chemical messengers. There is a great deal of similarity between the functions of nervous and endocrine systems. However, compared to the nervous system, the endocrine system is much slower to act but its influence lasts much longer.
[4] It comes as a surprise but it is true that the gut has more nerve cells than the spinal cord.
[5] It also makes the stomach secrete its juice but we don't see it.

aspects of the lifestyle which have not been discussed in detail in previous chapters.

We deal directly with our guts when we eat, and when we evacuate. We have little control over what goes on between these two events.

Eating

For a healthy gut, the way we eat is as important as what we eat. Some important aspects of eating have been discussed below.

When should we eat?

The simple answer is: eat only when hungry. This is possible if the meals are not very heavy, and there is no nibbling and munching between meals.

Where do we eat?

Eat in a peaceful atmosphere. Peace within and peace without are important for good digestion.

What to eat?

Eat a wholesome balanced diet. What constitutes such a diet has been discussed in Chapter 3. For easy digestion, and for avoiding problems like gas, some spices are very helpful. Modern medicine is only beginning to understand and acknowledge the value of spices. But fortunately some of the understanding which Ayurveda had about spices has survived in our culinary practices. Ginger (*adrak*), turmeric (*haldi*), coriander (*dhania*), mint (*pudina*) and fenugreek (*methi*), apart from being a concentrated supply of antioxidants, help prevent flatulence by facilitating digestion. Further, the food should be freshly cooked. It may be possible to prevent gross spoilage by refrigeration, but refrigerated food is likely to contribute to flatulence. The reason is that cold storage converts some of the starch in food into resistant starch. Resistant starch does not get digested by the digestive juices. Therefore, it reaches the large intestine, where it is fermented by bacteria. Fermentation results in the formation of gases, which in turn leads to flatulence.

How much should we eat?

A brief answer would be: neither too much, nor too little. The dictum in Ayurveda is to imagine that the stomach has four compartments: fill one part with water, two parts with food, and leave one part empty. In other words, at the end of a meal one should not be so full that it is impossible to eat any more. Regarding the distribution of food between meals, it is recommended that the largest meal of the day should be lunch. One may have two more meals – breakfast and dinner – and they should both be light. Eating between meals should be limited, if at all, and should be restricted to a fruit, a light snack or a healthy drink.

How do we eat?

One should always sit down to eat, preferably with the rest of the family. Whether it is with the family or colleagues, a small mismatch in timings should not be allowed to come in way of starting the meal together. Having settled down to eat, one should pray before eating. The prayer may be loud and collective, or silent and individual, but is important to remind us of the true significance of food. In yoga, food is a part of physical culture.[6] Physical culture is designed to keep the body healthy. The body should be healthy because it is our instrument of action. If our instrument is not in good shape, the action cannot be satisfactory. Action should be not just satisfactory, but the best that we are capable of because it has to be fit to be offered to the Divine, whose instruments we are. It is also by the divine grace that we receive and digest the food, and it is to the Divine in us that the food has to be offered. Reminding ourselves of these subtleties

---

[6] The other major components of physical culture are exercise and sleep.

at every meal is important because, being frail creatures given to sensory pleasures, we are likely to be carried away by many irrelevant considerations while eating. If we treat food as a sensory pleasure, we would select what tastes good; and if we get what we like, we would eat more than we should out of greed. On the other hand, if we realise the true purpose of food, we would select what is good for the body, eat just the right amount – neither too much nor too little, and still enjoy the meal. In short, with the right attitude to food, what is good (*shreyas*) also becomes pleasant (*preyas*). We enjoy the meal irrespective of its taste. We should retain the appreciation of good taste, but we should not be attached to good taste. Our happiness at mealtimes is no longer dependent on getting food that tastes good, and getting lots of it. By overcoming this dependence, we secure freedom – a freedom which ensures happiness which is independent of what we get to eat. This happiness is part of the bliss which is independent of external circumstances. The *Isha Upanishad* says in its first verse, 'renounce and enjoy' (*tena tyaktena bhunjitha*). Apparently it is contradictory: how can we do both – renounce and enjoy. But the renunciation referred to here is the inner renunciation, and inward detachment. In fact, we can truly enjoy the world only if we have renounced it from within. Because, with inner renunciation, we are not plagued by the fear how long the pleasure will last – we are not dependent on the pleasure for our happiness. Our happiness comes not from fleeting pleasures but from a source that is truly constant and dependable.

Having said the prayer, eat slowly. If you have got into the habit of eating fast, you should put the spoon down on the plate after each morsel. Relish each morsel as a marvel of nature – in fact, not one but several marvels. The way a plant grows capturing simple substances from the soil and air, and energy from sunlight, and the way our body digests the plants to get back the energy and raw materials of life involves a long series of highly organised and original feats of creative chemistry.

What should one do after eating?

End the meal with a prayer, and follow it up with a few minutes of rest. If you have a weak digestive system, you may sit for a few minutes in the *vajrasana* posture. Then move about slowly, may be in the house itself, for about ten minutes. How about 'an after-dinner walk'? It is not proper to take a brisk walk after any meal. If a person has a heart disease, it can even be dangerous to take any exercise after a meal. The reason is that digestion needs additional blood flow to the gut. On the other hand, exercise needs additional blood flow to the muscles. Creating a situation in which two regions of the body need extra blood flow simultaneously is dangerous for the heart. Hence a walk, either after breakfast, or after dinner, should be a slow one. It is better not to walk at all, after lunch, specially during hot weather. The reason is that exposure to heat increases blood flow to the skin (to increase the heat loss from the body). To increase blood flow to three regions simultaneously (gut, muscles and skin) can be disastrous for a weak heart. After lunch, it is best to rest sitting down (in *vajrasana* or otherwise) and then lie down – flat on the back, or on the left side – for about half an hour. If one wants to sleep after lunch, the nap should be just about an hour, not longer. Lying down after lunch has a significance that goes beyond digestion and sleep – it is also a good preventive for back aches.

What are the incorrect ways of eating?

A few don'ts in relation to eating: do not eat in a state of agitation or anger; eat only after settling down in a peaceful mood. Avoid multi-tasking while eating. Eating needs all your attention. In the long run it does not pay to save time by eating while walking or driving. Avoid talking while eating too. A little friendly conversation is alright, but mealtime is not the time for serious arguments. Avoid cold foods like ice cream, and cold drinks. Cold food and drinks slow down digestion. Finally, do not take a brisk walk or any other heavy exercise immediately after meals. The ideal interval between meals and exercise is at least four hours.

Evacuation

Evacuation once a day is generally not a problem for a mentally relaxed person with a good diet and regular physical activity. One should establish the routine of emptying the bowels at roughly the same time everyday – early morning is probably the best; at least it is the most convenient. It is helpful to take one or two glasses of water (at room temperature, or warm – but not cold) before going to the toilet. Spend at least five minutes on the toilet seat, but not more than fifteen. The bowel movement should begin within this interval. If it does not, do not strain, and do not worry. Just take a spoon or two of ispaghula husk (*isabgol*) at breakfast; more of this later when we discuss constipation. Constipation should not be neglected, but at the same time it is not proper to be obsessed with once-a-day evacuation. Neither the failure to relieve oneself once in a while, nor evacuating twice on some days is a serious matter. The gut is like a child: too much of attention makes it turn difficult.

Other lifestyle factors

Although the focus in this chapter is on diet and eating, the gut does not live in isolation. Its health depends also on other lifestyle factors such as regular physical activity, adequate sleep, and mental peace.

THE MISBEHAVING GUT

Discussing all the disorders of the gut is beyond the scope of this book. A few disorders which have a specially intimate relationship with the lifestyle have been discussed below.

Irritable bowel syndrome

Irritable bowel syndrome (IBS) is the commonest disorder in gastroenterology practice.[7] It is a chronic condition, and therefore the same patient keeps visiting the doctor repeatedly for years. If he gets tired of one doctor, he goes to another. But he may still not get cured because the doctor alone cannot fix the condition. The patient gets cured only when he takes charge of his own health, and changes his life and the way he looks at life. The symptoms are not constant; they change from time to time. The disease is not constant; it keeps going away and coming back. But it does not have to keep coming back: it leaves permanently when the patient gives it a befitting farewell.

Symptoms

A change in bowel habits apparently without any rhyme or reason should alert a person to the possibility of IBS. The change may be towards constipation or loose motions. Thus IBS may be either constipation-predominant or diarrhoea-predominant, and the dominant symptom may change with time even in the same person. There may be abdominal pain, usually in the lower abdomen, which may be described as colicky pain (rising and falling intermittently) or cramps (constant and severe pain). Another troublesome symptom is distension, which usually worsens as the day progresses. Both pain and distension are relieved temporarily upon relieving oneself. But, the person may not be really 'satisfied': he may have a feeling of incomplete evacuation. Some patients having IBS sometimes have mucus in the stool, but never blood. Blood in the stool should alert the person to something more serious than IBS, something that needs urgent medical attention.

[7.] IBS is quite different from IBD (Inflammatory Bowel Disease). While IBD also has a psychological component, it is a much more serious disorder than IBS

What causes IBS?

Although IBS gives a lot of trouble that goes on for long periods, there is hardly any abnormality that can be found in the gut on clinical examination or even after sophisticated investigations such as endoscopy, X-rays or ultrasound. IBS is the bodily manifestation of an underlying mental distress. It does not mean that those who have IBS are specially unfortunate in having more than their share of problems in life. Rather, it is the reaction of these persons to their problems which creates the distress. Nobody's life is perfect, nobody is completely satisfied with life as it is. But some people have a tendency to react negatively to unpleasant events and circumstances than is warranted. They get unduly anxious and worried about everything. Chronic worry eventually shows up as physical symptoms. What the physical symptoms are depends on the weak points in the body. The weak points depend to a large extent on heredity. Thus with the same amount of stress one person may get high blood pressure, another migraine, and yet another IBS. What is inherited, however, is only the tendency to get a particular disease. Whether a person actually gets it, and how badly he is affected by it, can be modified greatly by the way the person reacts to the ups and downs of life. The same person may also have a tendency to get more than one disease. That is why IBS is often associated with other ailments rooted in mental stress such as headaches or sleeplessness.

Managing IBS

IBS is often considered incurable but this is not necessarily true. By going to its root cause and correcting it, one can more or less eliminate its symptoms. With even a greater certainty, one can be free from the misery associated with symptoms of IBS.

Gut hygiene

The when, where, what, how, etc of eating discussed earlier is known as gut hygiene. While it is good for everyone to practise the hygiene, it is specially important for those suffering from IBS.

Managing constipation and diarrhoea

While constipation and diarrhoea are a nuisance, they are not a serious threat. Fortunately both improve with a higher fibre intake. To supplement the fibre intake further, *isabgol* is very useful. For constipation one may have *isabgol* with water, milk or curd. For diarrhoea, it is best to have *isabgol* with some curd. In either case, the dose is 1-2 teaspoons of *isabgol* once or twice a day, followed by at least one glass of water. The water is important so that *isabgol* has enough water available to soak, and it can form a viscous mass. It helps constipation by increasing the bulk of the residue in the large intestine. *Isabgol* also helps diarrhoea by binding the stool. Thus *isabgol* normalises gut motility: it reduces the motility of the gut which moves too much, and increases the mobility of the sluggish one. Constipation may also exist independent of IBS, and we shall return to it again.

Positive thinking

There is no problem in life which cannot be viewed positively. IBS itself has some positive features: it is a mild, manageable disease; it is inconvenient but not life-threatening, it is not associated with a structural lesion of the gut such as ulceration; and it does not predispose one to more serious ailments such as cancer.

Let go

Persons with IBS are usually obsessed with the body. They take notice of the slightest changes in bodily function, worry about these changes, and start imagining their worst implications and consequences. Chronic self-absorption of any type is a torture. To some extent one has to let go. A lot of things, including the gut, can take good care of themselves.

This might seem contradictory to the general tenor of this book. The reader has been encouraged throughout to sharpen his awareness of the body. But there is a difference between the sensitivity that is healthy, and one that may lead to conditions like IBS. It is certainly desirable to sensitise the consciousness of the body so that one knows when something is wrong. But there should also be an admiration for the wonder that the body is, and the confidence that the self-healing mechanisms of the body will correct whatever is wrong. Instead, the person with IBS adds to his perception of the body an imagination that predicts the worst. In short, the person with IBS should replace pessimistic awareness by an optimistic awareness of the body. Further, the optimism is based on facts, and is therefore fully justified.

Meditation

Meditation gives the inner silence which is required for reflection, introspection and reorientation. The resolutions arrived at during meditation facilitate the attitudinal changes required for getting better.

Visualisation

Towards the end of meditation, about five minutes may be spent on visualisation. Imagine a group of school children running about noisily in the playground. The sports teacher arrives and blows a whistle. The children quickly form lines. After a few minutes, they are swinging gracefully in tune with the beat of music. What a spectacular PT display! Transfer this analogy to the gut. Your gut right now is like the disorganised bunch of school children. Imagine that the Divine blows a whistle. The gut starts getting organised and moving gracefully and rhythmically. This transformation corresponds to self-healing, which the Divine has built into bodily functions. Visualise the corrective transformation of your gut three or four times a day, for about five minutes.

Music

Sweet and slow, soothing instrumental music is a good background for meditation and visualisation. Even otherwise, listening to slow music has a remarkable relaxing effect on the mind-body complex.

Constipation

Not everyone who thinks he is constipated is truly so. The really valid indicator of constipation is hard stool. Failure to relieve oneself everyday is not constipation unless the stool is hard. Constipation can be really obstinate. However, treating from every angle which may be possibly responsible for perpetuating it, it is generally possible to get rid of it.

Treatment

The first remedy that should be tried is to improve the diet. It is often effective by itself. If that is not enough, other measures may be added.

<u>Diet</u>

The dietary fibre intake should be increased and this can be done by:
  a. Consuming whole cereals such as brown rice, whole wheat flour, and pulses with the seed coat intact (*sabut dal*)
  b. Increasing the fruit and vegetable intake: the ideal is to have 5-6 helpings per day. A few specific fruits such as papaya and grapes have a mild laxative effect due to constituents other than dietary fibre. If that does not work, the fibre intake may be further increased by taking 1-2 teaspoonfuls of *isabgol* once or twice a day. Leave the isabgol husk in a small quantity of water in a kalori for about 5 minutes. Eat up the isabgol and follow it up with at least one glass of water. The water ensures that the isabgol would be able to swell up in the stomach and do a good job as a bulking agent.

A HIGH FIBRE DIET

Consume	Avoid
Whole wheat flour	Refined wheat flour (Maida)
Brown bread	White bread
Brown rice	White rice
Whole pulses	Dehusked pulses
Vegetables	Sago
Fruits (with the skin and seeds, if possible)	Arrowroot

Fluid intake
Increasing the water intake helps ease of constipation. A glass of warm water taken in the morning just before going to the toilet facilitates bowel movement.

Exercise
Regular physical activity is an integral part of a healthy lifestyle. For the constipated person, there is an additional incentive for taking exercise regularly as it helps regular bowel movement.

Let go
Psychologists have a theory that holding on to the stool reflects the attitude of the constipated person to hold on to every grievance in life. Be that as it may, it is much better to forgive, forget and be merry than to keep sulking. By refusing to forgive, the person whom we punish the most is ourselves. The 'take it easy' attitude makes it easier to deal with constipation.

No laxatives
Contrary to commonsense, laxatives actually perpetuate constipation. It happens because in a normal case we empty only a small length of the large intestine (Fig. 14.3). Laxatives stimulate the mobility of the large intestine and empty out a much longer length. The result is that now it needs time (may be two days or more) for the large intestine to fill up enough to create an urge for defecation. During these two days the person gets all the more convinced that he has a very obstinate constipation. If he does not have the patience to wait for 2-3 days, he takes another dose of the laxative. The laxative leads to a motion alright, but at the expense of emptying too much of the bowels. The result is another bout of constipation until enough of faecal matter has collected. Thus the laxative itself becomes the cause of the constipation. The way out is to wait for 2-3 days patiently. Relax: what is inside must come out one day – there is nowhere else it can go. However, during this waiting period, the large intestine gets time to absorb more and more water from whatever stool it contains. The result is a very hard stool, which is really the bad part of constipation. To prevent the stool from hardening, *isabgol* should

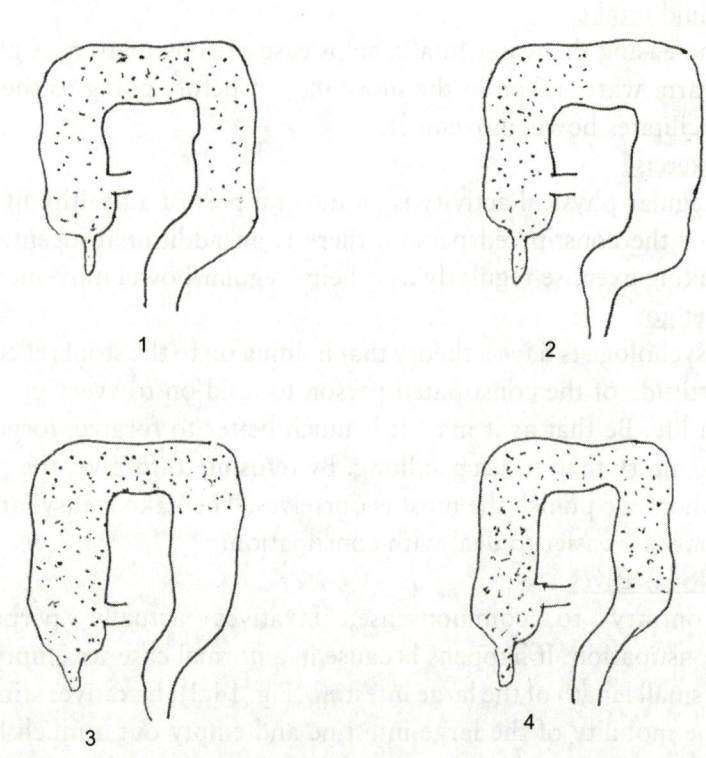

Fig. 14.3. Laxatives perpetuate constipation by emptying out too long a segment of the large intestine. Normally, when we pass a motion, we empty out only a small bit of the large intestine (1). The emptied part fills up again in a day or two, and then we get the urge to pass a motion again. Laxatives empty out much more of the large intestine (2). The day after the laxative (3), and even two days after the laxative (4), the intestine is still not full enough to create the urge for evacuation. What is needed is patience for the intestine to sufficiently fill up sufficiently. Taking a laxative at stage 3 or 4 will bring a motion, but once again the intestine will become as at 2, and will take several days to fill up adequately for creating the urge to evacuate.

(Based on Bijlani R., *Hum Kya Khayen* (Hindi). New Delhi: National Council of Educational Research and Training, 1989, Fig. 7.1.)

be had everyday during the 'waiting period'. However, it is best not to take any laxatives so that there are no waiting periods.[8]

<u>Do not strain</u>
In constipation, there is a natural tendency to strain. Straining regularly over years eventually leads to complications such as anal fissures, piles and varicose veins. To prevent these complications, one should never strain. To achieve this ideal, the following graded approach may be used:

a. Prevent constipation – that is the best.
b. Treat constipation as discussed already.
c. If unsuccessful, have patience. Have *isabgol*, but do not strain.
d. Relax. Be happy the day you complete your ablutions. Stay happy the day you do not. Just spend 5-10 minutes in the toilet, and leave it happy irrespective of the outcome[9]. If you are unable to perform the ablutions, take a spoon or two of *isabgol* at breakfast. Follow it up up with at least one glass of water.
e. If you feel an urge to empty your bbwels, but are unable to do so because the stool is too hard, *do not strain*. Apply some oil (may be, mustard oil) on your finger and lubricate the anal passage. By gentle rounded motions, gradually the anus will open up and you will be able to work your way up through the anus. Keep applying more oil to the finger periodically. Finally, you will be able to touch the hard stool. Manipulate the stool with the finger. Mould it by pressing it from different directions. Break it with the oily finger into a few pieces. Now you will find it

---

[8] *Isbagol* is not a laxative. It is a dietary supplement. It facilitates a motion by making the stool bulkier and softer. It does not rush the large intestine to empty out an unduly large amount.

[9] I can leave the toilet happy even if I have spent fifteen minutes there with 'zero results' because I don't waste time there. I read while on the toilet seat.

will be easy to pass the motion without straining.
f. The last resort. In the very, very rare eventuality of none of the above approaches working, contact your doctor who may give you an enema.

Acidity, Gastritis and Peptic Ulcer

These are three related conditions of increasing severity. During acidity, there is just increased production of acid in the stomach. In gastritis, the increased acid production goes on long enough to make the surface of the stomach inflamed. In case of a peptic ulcer, the damage to the stomach progresses to a level where a circular patch in the wall of the stomach erodes leading to the formation of a 'crater'. However, the basic defect in all these conditions is not necessarily the increased production of acid. More accurately, the defect is an imbalance between the acid, and the mechanisms which normally protect the stomach from the effects of the acid. Thus the cause of this cluster of diseases may be increased acid production, or weak protection, or both. That is why some people may produce more acid but have no problem whereas some others may have a problem even with normal acid production.

Underlying causes

Increased acid production or poor protection are the end result of several years of living a faulty lifestyle. Irregular meals, too much of chilli, eating in a hurry, smoking, drinking and mental stress are some of the better-known culprits. A typical patient having a peptic ulcer is ambitious, self-opinionated, wrapped up in himself, pessimistic, anxious, worried, hostile, lonely, and lacks love and intimacy in his relationships. He may have a stressful job involving night shifts.

Helicobacter pylori

Helicobacter pylori is the name of a germ that is often present in the stomachs of those having gastritis and peptic ulcers. Its relationship with these disorders is similar to that of acid. Many people harbour the germ without any problem, and a few may have the problem but not the germ in the stomach. However, in those having the problem, it is worthwhile testing for the presence of the germ, and eliminating it if it is there.

Treatment

Meals should be small, and a little more frequent than normal. It is better not to observe a fast or skip a meal because it is undesirable to let the acid act on an empty stomach – at least the acid should have some food to work on. Items which increase acid production should be avoided: these include chillies, tea, coffee, alcohol and smoking. One should change one's attitude to other people, events and circumstances in order to reduce mental stress.

If necessary, medication may be added to the above measures. A variety of antacids and drugs which reduce acid production are available but these should be used only under medical supervision. Your doctor may also decide to eliminate Helicobacter pylori by giving suitable drugs. Drug therapy of acid-peptic disease has progressed so much in the last few decades that surgery is almost never needed.

Meditation and visualisation

Towards the end of a session of meditation, about five minutes may be spent on visualisation. First visualise your stomach with an inside surface which is an angry red and is pouring out acid. Then visualise it changing to a pleasing pink colour, like that of the petal of a pink rose. The acid is also gone now; there are just a few drops of dew. Focus your attention on the pink petal-like surface with a few glistening dew drops resting peacefully on it. Repeat the visualisation 3-4 times a day.

Yogic practices

It is more important to know what should not be done than what may be done. A person having acidity, gastritis or peptic ulcer should not do *pashchimuttanasana, yoga mudra* and *shashankasana*. Other yogic practices are permissible. Special attention may be paid to a few practices mentioned later in this chapter. *Vamana dhouti/kunjal* may be particularly helpful in acid-peptic disease but should be done only under expert guidance and supervision.

Gas

Gas in the gut may be either in the stomach or in the large intestine: both are entirely different and therefore merit separate treatment.

Gas in the stomach

The origin of gas in the stomach is the air that has been swallowed with food. The swallowed air causes eructation, which continues till the air has been belched out. If one eats properly, not much of air should get swallowed. Air gets swallowed when we eat in a hurry, or talk while eating, and keep the mouth open while chewing. All these things happen more often in a person who is mentally stressed. The treatment is obvious: manage the stress, eat slowly, do not talk while eating, and keep the mouth closed while chewing. In addition, it also helps to avoid tea, coffee, chocolate, orange juice, peppermint, too much fat and alcohol in the diet.

Gas in the large intestine

Gas in the large intestine is generated by the fermentation of undigested and indigestible food material. The gas so produced is expelled as flatus. Everybody produces some gas in the large intestine. Therefore, up to a point, flatus is as normal as breathing. However, difficulty arises when the amount of flatus increases to an abnormal level. Since flatus results from an interaction between food and germs, its treatment involves paying attention to both.

Some foods, such as beans, specially kidney beans (*rajmah*), chick peas (*chane*) and black gram (*urad*), tend to be flatulent. Mung beans (*moong*) and lentils (*masoor*) are much better in this respect. Some foods specifically prevent flatulence, eg spices such as ginger (*adrak/saunth*), omum (*ajwan*), aniseed (*saunf*), and asafetida (*hing*).

Some people cannot digest milk and therefore drinking milk gives them flatulence. They should avoid milk. However, they may take some milk in tea, and they are able to tolerate curd. Unripe banana and food stored in the refrigerator may also give flatulence.

Regarding bacteria, curd (yogurt) is a good way of introducing into the gut bacteria which produce less flatulence. Eating more curd leads to a competition between its bacteria and flatulence-producing germs for a limited amount of food in the large intestine. Thus the better bacteria in curd drive out the flatulence-producing germs. That is how curd helps reduce flatulence. In contrast with curd, a high fat or a high protein diet promotes the growth of gems which lead to flatulence. This is specially true of protein in non-vegetarian foods. Therefore these items should be avoided.

YOGIC PRACTICES FOR GASTROINTESTINAL DISORDERS

The person who has problems with the gut should also attend to the rest of the body and he should perform the same set of yogic practices as anybody else, except for the practices which might harm him. However, there are a few practices recommended by Swami Vivekananda Kendra, Bangalore, which are particularly useful for normalising gastrointestinal functions: these have been listed below:

Asanas

Pavanmuktasana, Uttanapadasana, Naukasana, Bhujangasana, Shalabhasana, Dhanurasana, Trikonasana and Katichakrasana.

Pranayama

As in Chapter 1, except that a person having hernia **should not** practise *kapalabhati*.

Uddiyana bandha

Stand with the feet apart, bend down a little at the waist, place the palms on the thighs and press a little. Keep the arms straight.

Then breathe out completely through the mouth. Use the abdominal muscles to empty the lungs. Press the hands against the thighs. Tighten the upper part of the body and suck in the abdomen. Hold the body in this position as long as possible. Then breathe in slowly. Relax the abdomen and rise up to the standing posture.

Agnisara and *nauli* are advanced practices based on the *uddiyana bandha*, and can be helpful in some gastrointestinal disorders. But for learning any of these physical practices, personal instruction and guidance are essential.

Meditation and Visualisation

As described for individual disorders above.

Special techniques

Techniques such as *vamana dhouti/kunjal, shankhaprakshalana/ laghushankhaprakshalana* should be done only under expert guidance and supervision, if at all. In most cases, they should not be necessary.

CLOSING THOUGHTS

The best guts are those that are the least cared for: there is a grain of truth in this adage. People with gastrointestinal problems often **have** their attention all focused on the body, specially the gut.

This may happen particularly in old age with those who do not have much to do. Getting busy with interesting activities often settles down the gut.

Frequently Asked Questions

What is the best time to have water in relation to meals?

There is general agreement on the following two rather similar dictums:
   a. One should not have too much water along with a meal; it may dilute the digestive juices and reduce their activity. Up to one glass is considered acceptable. There is no harm in having no water at all with the meals.
   b. One should not have water during the meals.

There is no agreement on whether water should be taken before meals or after meals. It is possible to support both on logical grounds. Having water before the meals helps avoid overeating. Having water after the meals acts as a partial mouthwash and thereby aids dental hygiene. The choice may be made depending on whether or not it is possible to rinse the mouth. Taking water during the meals can also be justified. If water is taken just before shifting from one food item to the other, the water helps in rinsing the mouth, thereby preventing a mix-up of tastes. Wanting to accentuate sensory pleasure is not a yogic reason, but is a reason all the same. The key point is to avoid taking more than one glass of water during a meal.

FOR FURTHER READING

Bijlani R.L., *Nutrition: a practical approach*. New Delhi: Jaypee, 2nd Edition, 2007.
Chopra D., *Perfect Digestion*, London: Rider/Random, 1995.
Nagarathna R, Nagendra HR. *Yoga for Digestive Disrorders*, **Bangalore: Swami Vivekananda Yoga Prakashana, 2002.**

Appendix 1

Yogic Practices for Lifestyle Disorders

1. Contrary to what the patients often think, and demand, individual asanas are not specific for the treatment of a particular disorder. An increase in physical activity, an improvement in the flexibility of the body, and a calming effect on the mind are non-specific effects of all asanas, and are the major contributors to the improvement observed in a wide range of disorders.
2. The specificity, even if it existed, is not that important because we should be concerned not just with the immediate physical ailment: it is sensible to be interested in improving the health and fitness of the whole body.
3. Since most of the people looking at yoga for the treatment of a lifestyle disorder are likely to be past youth, strenuous practices have been omitted from the list given here.
4. It is more important to know which asanas to avoid than to know which specific ones to do for a particular ailment. Therefore, that information has been included here.
5. For diagrams and some details of the practices, please see Chapter 1.

WARMING UP
Loosening exercises
Loosening of the fingers, wrists, elbows, shoulders, hips and knees[1]
Neck rotations[2]

Breathing exercises
Hands in and out breathing, Hand stretch breathing, Ankle stretch breathing, Forward and backward bending synchronised with breathing[3]

ASANAS
Lying down postures
Shavasana
Prishthbhoomi tadasana
Setubandhasana
Pavanmuktasana
Shavasana

Sitting postures
Pashchimottanasana[4]
Konasana[5]
Shavasana
Vajrasana
Shashankasana

---

[1] Specially important for those having arthritis.
[2] Specially important for those engaged in desk work. Those having cervical spondylosis should not do clockwise and anti-clockwise rotation of the neck.
[3] Specially important for those having bronchial asthma.
[4] Should be avoided by those having back pain or neck pain; good for those having constipation.
[5] Should be avoided by those having coronary heart disease, specially if they have had a recent major problem.

Ushtrasana[6]
Parvatasana

Lying down (prone) postures
Makarasana
Bhujangasana[7]
Makarasana
Dhanurasana or Shalabhasana[8]
Makarasana

Standing postures
Tadasana
Padahastasana[9]
Tadasana
Trikonasana
Katichakrasana
Shavasana

PRANAYAMAS
Full yogic breathing[10]

---

[6] Should not be done by those having hernia, severe high blood pressure, low back pain, and by those who have undergone recent abdominal or chest surgery.

[7] Specially important for those having back pain, but should be avoided by those having neck pain; should not be done by those who have undergone abdominal surgery within the last two months; helps bronchial asthma.

[8] Specially recommended for diabetes and digestive disorders; *shalabhasana* is easier than *dhanurasana*.

[9] Should be avoided by those having back pain, neck pain, vertigo or severe high blood pressure; helps constipation, improves digestion, helps menstrual problems.

[10] Helps restore peace if angry or exhausted.

Kapalabhati[11]
Nadi shuddhi pranayama
Cooling pranayama[12]
Bhramari[13]

MEDITATION[14]

---

[11] Should not be done by those having epilepsy, vertigo, hernia, peptic ulcer, high blood pressure, coronary heart disease, back pain, or neck pain (cervical spondylosis); helps breathing problems and digestive problems.

[12] Specially recommended for high blood pressure and nasobronchial allergies. Should not be done if the person has a cold or sore throat, or if the weather is cold or damp.

[13] Improves the voice, and therefore specially recommended for singers; also good for mental stress, anger and high blood pressure.

[14] Specially recommended for mental stress and high blood pressure.

Appendix 2

Words of Wisdom

It should take long for self-cure to replace medicine, because of the fear, self-distrust and unnatural physical reliance on drugs which medical science has taught to our minds and bodies and made our second nature.

—Sri Aurobindo

Human body, the living temple of God, and a living miraculous machine, is self-reliant in maintaining health as well as curing ill health through the natural medicines produced in its own factory.

—Mahatma Gandhi

The man who can forgive is doing all those around him, and especially himself, a huge favour.

—Benjamin Stein

Though no one can go back and make a brand new beginning, anyone can start from now and make a brand new end.

—Anonymous

It is better to live as long as you want rather than want as long as you live.

—Socrates

We are all perfectly imperfect.
— Dr Bernie Siegel

One should not eat in order to please the palate, but just to keep the body going. When each organ of sense subserves the body, and through the body the soul, its special relish disappears and then alone does it begin to function in the way nature intended it to.
— Mahatma Gandhi

I love to sleep. It's really the best of both worlds. You get to be alive and unconscious.
— Rita Rudner

Unappalled by the fear of death canst thou leave to Him, not as an experiment, with a calm and entire faith thy ailments? Thou shalt find that in the end He exceeds the skill of a million doctors.
— Sri Aurobindo

Establish a greater peace and quietness in your body; that will give you the strength to resist attacks of illness.
— The Mother (of Sri Aurobindo Ashram)

Knowledge always leads to love, and love to service.
— Mother Teresa

You are not fully dressed until you wear a smile on your face.
— Mahatma Gandhi

Laughter is a form of internal jogging.
— Norman Cousins

The grand essentials of happiness are: something to do, something to love, and something to hope for.
— Alan Chalmers

Disease thrives on pessimism
—SHELLEYS

While pessimists have a more accurate view of the world, optimists live a lot longer and have a better time.
—DR BERNIE SIEGEL

A narcissistic society that encourages such great expectations is bound to induce great disappointments.
—DR NICK READ

Yoga is not a way of giving up a little to get a lot. It is a way of giving up everything, wanting nothing, and getting everything.
—DR RAMESH BIJLANI

Stress is an ignorant state. It believes that everything is an emergency.
—NATALIE GOLDBERG

What goes on in a patient's mind is often the key to whether he will get well.
—DR CARL SIMONTON

The mind and body work together, with the body being the screen where the movie is shown.
—EVY MCDONALD

Worry is spiritual nearsightedness, a fumbling way of looking at little things, and of magnifying their value.
—ANNA ROBERTSON

Worry lives a long way from rational thought.
—MARY ROACH

You are only as sick as the secrets you keep. Flush these skeletons out of the closet and you will be healed.
— Dr Arthur Brownstein

It is more important to know what kind of a person has a disease than what kind of a disease a person has.
— Dr William Osler

Our mental attitudes affect first our susceptibility to disease, then our ability to overcome it.
— Dr Bernie Siegel

The living body is the best pharmacy ever devised.
— Dr Deepak Chopra

Drugs are not always necessary. Belief in recovery always is.
— Norman Cousins

If you are lucky enough to find a way of life you love, you have to find the courage to live it.
— John Irving

If scientists suddenly discovered a drug that was as powerful as love in creating health, it would be heralded as a medical breakthrough and marketed overnight – especially if it had as few side effects and was as inexpensive as love.
— Dr Larry Dossey

I believe the evidence is compelling: love and intimacy lead to greater health and healing, while loneliness and isolation predispose one to suffering, disease and premature death.
— Dr Dean Ornish

Meditation is based on the principle that clearing a clutter is enough for clarity to surface spontaneously.
— Dr Ramesh Bijlani